DCIS of the Breast
Taking Control

Professor John Boyages, MD, PhD

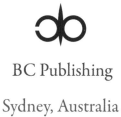

BC Publishing

Sydney, Australia

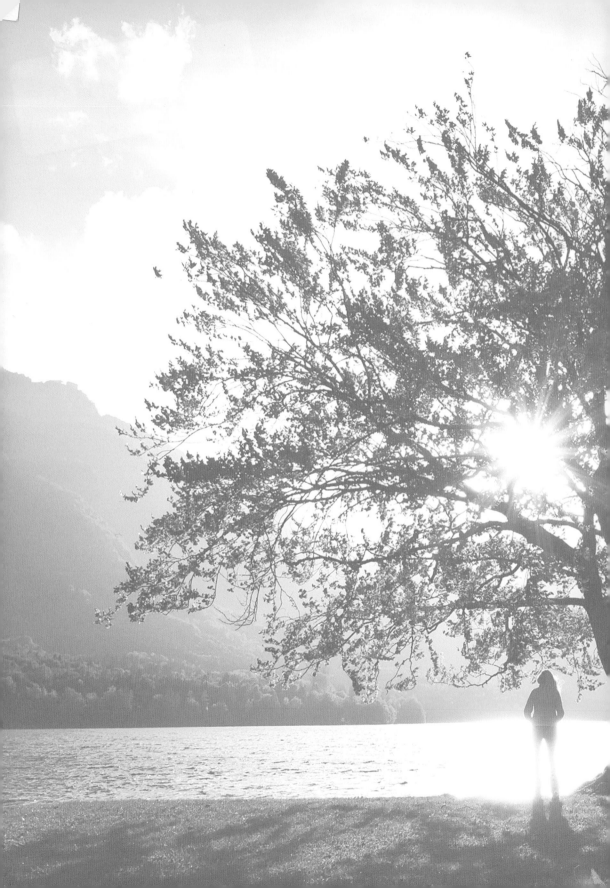

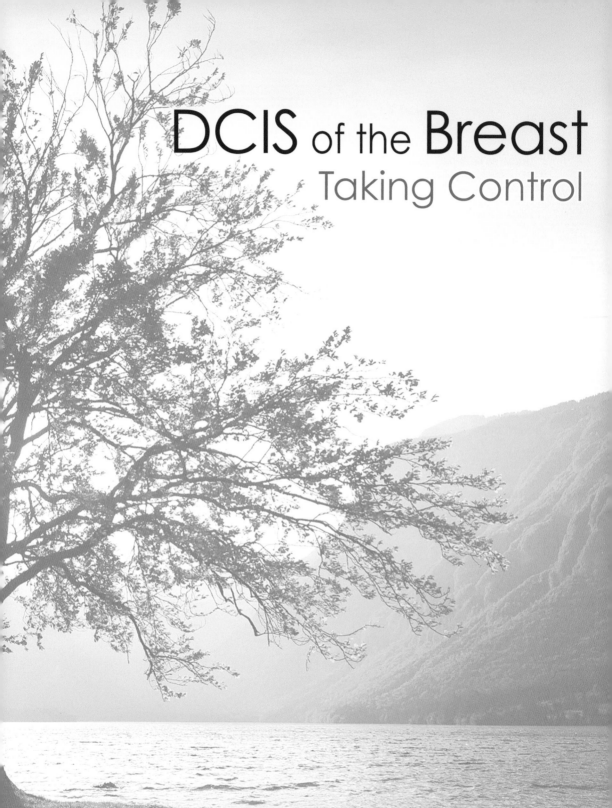

DCIS of the Breast
Taking Control

Professor John Boyages, MD, PhD

DCIS of the Breast: Taking Control
BC Publishing, Australia
PO Box 568, Beecroft, NSW 2119, Australia
bcpublishers@gmail.com
bcpublish.com

First edition published 2014.
ISBN-13: 978-0-9806311-4-2 (Soft cover)

National Library of Australia Cataloguing-in-Publication entry: Book
Author: Boyages, John.
Title: DCIS of the Breast: Taking Control / John Boyages.
Edition: 1st ed.
ISBN: 978-0-9806311-4-2
Subjects:
Breast--Precancerous conditions.
Breast--Cancer--Treatment.
Breast--Cancer--Diagnosis.
Dewey Number: 616.99449

DEDICATION

To the brave patients dealing with the dilemmas of DCIS of the breast.
To Dianne, thank you for all your love, humor and extraordinary support.

PRAISE FOR *DCIS OF THE BREAST: TAKING CONTROL*

DCIS of the Breast: Taking Control covers the complicated subject of DCIS in plain English and includes some of the latest diagnostic and treatment techniques we are now offering our patients including oncoplastic surgery.

—Dr James French
Head of Breast Surgery
Westmead Breast Cancer Institute

Nobody wants to hear the words "You have DCIS," but Professor John Boyages has helped many women not just survive but thrive after the heartbreak of a diagnosis of DCIS or breast cancer. John's first book, *Breast Cancer: Taking Control* set a high standard and this book has filled an important gap. Apart from his clinical work, he is also a passionate advocate for breast cancer education, and whenever journalists need help with a breast cancer story, he responds promptly without medical gobbledygook! John has won several awards for services to medicine and the media, and the tips in this book are a must-read for anyone with diagnosed or suspected DCIS.

—Jane Worthington
Health reporter
Woman's Day, Reader's Digest HealthSmart and *The Sunday Telegraph*

Dr John Boyages is a leader amongst his peers, has a strong sense of duty and is committed to professionalism. John is an extremely knowledgeable and technically skilled physician, best characterized by his commitment to comprehensive and compassionate patient care. This exciting book provides clear, understandable solutions that put the reader at ease; it is an excellent and invaluable resource for patients and caregivers and a first-rate addition to the oncology, sexual medicine, and cancer survivorship fields.

—Michael L. Krychman, MD
Executive Director of the Southern California Center for Sexual Health and Survivorship Medicine, Associate Clinical Professor and Director of Ann's High Risk Breast Ovarian Center, University of California, Irvine

DCIS of the Breast: Taking Control is a must-read for patients who not only have just been diagnosed with DCIS but also those who were treated in the past. John highlights the multidisciplinary approach and reviews the entire spectrum of patient care, from diagnosis, deciding on the best option, treatment, post-treatment follow-up and survivorship issues.

Using his now familiar Control Points in twenty comprehensive yet concise chapters, this thorough, practical book is an essential clinical guide written for patients with DCIS and their families but also valuable for surgeons, oncologists, nurses, and general practitioners.

—Professor Owen Ung
Head of Breast and Endocrine unit
Royal Brisbane and Women's Hospital

This is a superb book for any patient, their family member or friend, with a diagnosis of DCIS of the breast. John is a great doctor who completed a fellowship with me at the Dana-Farber Cancer Institute in 1988. We advised many patients with DCIS from all over the world who were seeking second and third opinions at a time when little information was known and the disease became more common from screening mammography. In this book, John gives you his objective expert advice about all treatment options.

—Jay R. Harris, MD
Professor, Department of Radiation Oncology, Harvard Medical School
Chief, Radiation Oncology Department, Dana-Farber Cancer Institute

I'd be pleased to have John take care of any member of my own family, and if they had DCIS of the breast. I'd certainly recommend that they read this book—and I recommend it to you as well!"

—Daniel F. Hayes, MD
Stuart A. Padnos, Professor of Breast Cancer Research, University of Michigan

PRAISE FOR *BREAST CANCER: TAKING CONTROL*
(PUBLISHED 2010)

John Boyages is absolutely right: women do remember the first three months after initial diagnosis of breast cancer as the most confusing and frightening. I did. This is the first book to acknowledge and address that, and it is most welcome. This comprehensive yet personal guide will help women to feel that they can handle their [treatment] decisions because it gives them the information they need at the right time, and in one place.

—Sally Crossing, AM
Founding Chair, Breast Cancer Action Group NSW

An easy read for a layperson without a medical background—insightful and informative.

—Michelle Hanton OAM
Founder Dragons Abreast Australia

Dear John, I just got my hands on a copy of your new book. WOW! I couldn't put it down. What an absolutely brilliant book—unique, balanced, simple charts and yet quite detailed, empowering, compassionate and informative, informative, informative! WOW!

Congratulations. I'm sure women of Australia and beyond thank you.

—John Eden MD
Associate Professor of Reproductive Endocrinology University of NSW, Director Barbara Gross Research Unit and Sydney Menopause Centre, Royal Hospital for Women and Director Women's Health and Research Institute of Australia

FOREWORD

The diagnosis of ductal carcinoma in situ (DCIS) of the breast is a dilemma as its diagnosis can be difficult and treatment options confusing. Following a diagnosis of DCIS, many people today turn to the Internet to get answers before they see their doctor, but resources on the Web are often biased, inaccurate or unhelpful.

At long last, an international expert who has published widely on breast cancer and DCIS has written a book that focuses on what a patient needs to know from the point of diagnosis.

DCIS of the Breast: Taking Control takes you through all the critical "Control Points" after a diagnosis in a personal, plain English style, and in one place gives you all the information you need.

John Boyages is one of the world's leading radiation oncologists who not only treats patients with DCIS but continues to undertake research and lecture on this condition.

Thomas A. Buchholz, MD, FACR
Professor, Division of Radiation Oncology, The University of Texas MD Anderson Cancer Center, Houston, Texas and Fellow of the American Society of Radiation Oncology (FASTRO)

CONTENTS

PART 3: "MAINTAINING CONTROL"
TAKING CONTROL AFTER YOUR SURGERY

ABOUT THE AUTHOR

John Boyages, MB, BS (Hons), FRACR, PhD is a cancer specialist with over 30 years' experience in the diagnosis and treatment of breast cancer. He is now the Director and Professor of Breast Oncology at the Macquarie University Cancer Institute. He was the founding director of the Westmead Breast Cancer Institute from 1995 until 2011 and is also a busy clinician who cares for patients at Norwest Private and Genesis Cancer Care at the Macquarie University Hospitals.

Following his training at the University of Sydney and a fellowship at Harvard Medical School under the direction of Professor Jay Harris, he was appointed as a specialist radiation oncologist at Westmead Hospital in 1989. There, John founded one of the largest free breast cancer screening programs in the west of Sydney. In 1995, he won a grant to establish and direct the Westmead Breast Cancer Institute, which offers clinical care, research, education, and screening programs.

He has published more than 140 research and clinical articles and is committed to the dissemination of research findings to lay and professional audiences both nationally and internationally. John performs numerous national roles in his field, and his current international roles include: member of the International Union Against Cancer (UICC) for the Staging of Breast Cancer and member of the editorial board of the European Journal of Cancer. In 2006, John received a national Medical Media Award for outstanding service to the media and the community. In 2013, he was awarded a Rotary Vocational Excellence Award and was also a finalist in the NSW Australian of the Year. In 2014, he was awarded by AHEPA, The Ippokratis Award for outstanding achievement by a medical professional.

In 2010, John published his bestselling book for patients with cancer, *Breast Cancer: Taking Control*, which won the Foreword Reviews Book of the Year for Health in the same year. He is also the author of *Clinical Breast Examination: Taking Control*, a DVD for health professionals.

ACKNOWLEDGEMENTS

Firstly, thanks to all my friends, patients, neighbors, colleagues, and others who have helped by spurring me on to produce this work or giving me a lot of their precious time.

I would especially like to thank my wife, Dianne, for her ongoing patience and support and her understanding of the number of hours I spend away from our family pursuing my passion of helping women (and a few men) fight breast cancer and its precursor, DCIS. Thanks also to my beautiful children, Fiona and son-in-law David and grandson Jack, and Peter and daughter-in-law Lauren, for their ongoing humor, support, and understanding.

Expert medical review of sections of the book were undertaken by my colleagues, Professor Michael Bilous, Dr Deborah Cheung, Dr Elisabeth Elder, Dr Laura Essermen, Dr James French, Dr Jeremy Hsu, Dr Thomas Lam, Dr Kirsten Stuart, Dr Tim Wang, and A/Prof Nicholas Wilcken.

Special thanks to the book's Managing Editors, Jess Ní Chuinn and Fiona Richardson for project management and to Rachel Haimowitz, my U.S. editor, for her expert editing of this work.

Finally, thanks to my late father, Constantine, and mother, Fotini, who migrated from Greece after World War II and taught me the value of hard work, honesty, education, and lifelong learning, and for passing their values to all their children and grandchildren.

HOW TO USE THIS BOOK

This book is not a textbook about DCIS. It is a "behind the scenes" how-to book, designed to give you the key information you need at the twenty Control Points on your path to understand what DCIS means and how to ensure you and/or your family member gets the best advice and treatment.

Flow charts for the Control Points are found at the beginning of each chapter. Follow your possible paths and read the chapters that apply to your own situation. It's at these crossroads that you need the right information at the right time. In this book, there are three color themes used in the different parts as shown in the graphic below. Part 1, in red, is the time to "stop" and take stock of the situation, rather than rush into a decision you may regret. Part 2 is in orange as a lot of "caution" is required in this part of your journey. Some big decisions need to be made that can affect the rest of your life. Part 3 is in green, which means to "proceed with care" and details information you need to have at your fingertips after your surgery and when all your treatment is over.

The book includes real-life patient stories, key Web links, multiple figures and tables underpinned by an extensive Reference List. Glossary terms are in bold when used in text for the first time. Good luck in your journey, and I am sure that *DCIS of the Breast: Taking Control* will help you when life suddenly feels so out of control.

But remember, DCIS, properly treated, can have a nearly 100% success rate.

Part	Color	Action	Title	Taking Control	Control Points	Patient Stories
1	Red	STOP	Shock Control	Immediately after your diagnosis	3	8
2	Amber	CAUTION	Gaining Control	Before your surgery	7	3
3	Green	PROCEED WITH CARE	Maintaining Control	After your surgery	10	6

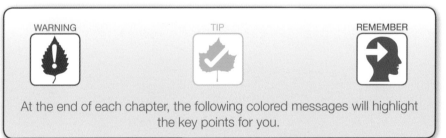

WARNING   TIP   REMEMBER

At the end of each chapter, the following colored messages will highlight the key points for you.

INTRODUCTION

Hi, my name is Professor John Boyages. I like my patients to call me John. Every week, I see at least 30–40 patients with breast cancer, either as a patient with a new diagnosis or for a checkup. About five patients I see every week have had a diagnosis of ductal carcinoma in situ, or **DCIS**.

My interest in breast cancer started back in 1983 when my mentor, Professor Allan Langlands, asked me to do some research with him during my training. After graduating from Sydney University with a degree in medicine and another in radiation oncology, I enrolled in a PhD and was invited to do further study at Harvard University. Since then, I have set up various programs in the west of Sydney and one in 2011 at the new Macquarie University Hospital. At Harvard, I worked with some of the best masters in the world. I am eternally grateful to leading MDs Jay Harris, Craig Henderson, Susan Love, Jim Connolly, Stuart Schnitt, Abe Recht, Dan Hayes and many others for allowing me to work with them at the Breast Evaluation Clinic (the "BEC") at the Dana-Farber Cancer Institute and the Beth Israel Hospital in Boston, and for helping me to learn good research practices and recognize good science.

My first real understanding of DCIS started in 1988 when I was invited by Dr Jay Harris to do a fellowship with him. Mammography was far more advanced back then in the United States than it was in Australia and I started seeing patients with this "new" disease called DCIS. Jay was seeing patient after patient for second and third opinions with DCIS. There was not a lot of information or studies done at that time, particularly about how to treat the disease without a **mastectomy** and we had to use our clinical judgment a lot of the time. We were seeing patients from all over the world. Patients had flown in from Paris, New York and from elsewhere in the U.S. to get the opinion from the master. I remember in one clinic a 35-year-old woman refused to have a mastectomy even though she had a very large area of DCIS, and an older patient who was a physician, with a tiny area of DCIS, for whom we recommended breast conservation just wanted her whole breast removed. Our clinic at the BEC was truly multidisciplinary with plastic surgeons, pathologists and radiologists helping the surgeons and radiation oncologists make the right decision for the individual patient.

By now, I have assumed you have been diagnosed with DCIS or have been told you most likely have DCIS. I presume you have had a **mammogram** that has shown some calcium spots or less frequently a small **density**. Perhaps you may have had a nipple rash or discharge. You may have had a core biopsy.

The aim of this book is to help you or your family member:

- understand what may happen after a diagnosis of non-invasive DCIS

- understand not only what treatments are available, but also how best to use them in your own situation

- understand the evidence supporting the treatment choices you may face after a diagnosis, including

  - Is what I have really DCIS?

  - Do I really need a mastectomy?

- Is breast conservation (removal of your DCIS, also known as a **lumpectomy**) the best approach for me?
- Can I get away without having radiotherapy?
- Do I need to check if the DCIS has progressed to invasive cancer and possibly spread to my lymph glands under my armpit?
- What are the side effects of all these treatments?
- Do I need hormonal treatment for my DCIS?
- What do I do if DCIS comes back?

• regain control by teaching you the evidence for treatment decisions and dispelling many myths.

This book will detail some of my insight and experience into what it's like to treat a patient who has just been diagnosed with DCIS. Sometimes, I find managing patients with DCIS somewhat harder than treating patients with invasive breast cancer. This is because there is often not one hard and fast answer and because there is diversity of opinion on the best approach.

There are many books and Web sites out there that will tell you what to do. I'll detail some of the best Web sites (and particularly Web links to specific information) throughout this book. I'm not going to repeat everything; I'll just give you the most important bits in a logical order. The trouble with Web sites and "support guides" is that they don't know what not to tell you. Basically, they give you too much information, and that can be pretty scary and difficult to sort through. Like in my first book, *Breast Cancer: Taking Control*, I will point out the important "Control Points" and guide you through this even more complicated garden maze.

One thing is certain: DCIS is a complex and often frustrating area that I will try to break down and explain for you in plain English. I will also provide key results from important medical publications about DCIS in easy-to-understand tables, lists and graphs. If you are not a data person, just skip over these and read only the text. I don't like rushing patients, so I go slowly through all of their questions. Everybody is different, of course—some women like to be told what to do, others like a moderate amount of information, and still others like a lot. Some people like copies of our peer-reviewed publications. One size doesn't fit all.

Remember, it's important not to rush into treatment. You have plenty of time to find a team that will look after you in the best possible way both physically and emotionally. It's best to get the right treatment the first time, even a month after your diagnosis, than to be rushed into making the wrong decision.

I will use many garden and other analogies in this book. When you look at a flower, like a rose, you will see the complexities of the petals wrapping around each other. The health-care system is also a complex maze, and in this book, using plain English examples often taken from nature, I will show you which turns to take so that you are taking control by always having the information you need at your fingertips.

Debbie's Story

I didn't sleep for a few days after I received a letter from my breast screening service saying I had to come back for more tests. I wasn't expecting to be told I had anything wrong. I took my friend with me and after two hours my breast felt worse for wear. I had more mammograms and a core biopsy. They said the area involved two parts of my breast. Another week wait! Back again and I'm told I had an "alphabet" rather than a diagnosis. What on earth was "DCIS"?

More waiting to see the surgeon who eventually recommended a mastectomy. Reconstruction was never discussed. I only found out about that later. I was very confused at first, feeling that they were removing my breast and it wasn't even cancer.

That was fifteen years ago. I had a reconstruction last year and a lift on the other side and I'm fine.

BE TREATED AS AN INDIVIDUAL

I constantly receive phone calls from friends, colleagues, or relatives who want advice about their individual situations. I decided that the only way to keep up with all of it was to write it down so that hopefully, others could learn from my experience. Since 1988, I have written about six publications specifically related to DCIS and have given countless lectures. One of them, written for the journal *Cancer*, is one of my most cited papers (Boyages et al. 1999). I still do a lot of second opinions about DCIS and feel that the early detection of DCIS through mammography has helped reduce the overall incidence of breast cancer. In the last five years, the incidence of real breast cancer (invasive disease) has dropped in many countries including the U.S. and Australia. In my view, this is partly due to women being a bit more careful in taking **hormone replacement therapy (HRT)** but also by finding DCIS that would have turned into invasive cancer had it not been detected earlier (Coombs et al. 2010).

There is no doubt about it: treating DCIS is controversial. There are different schools of thought. Some pathologists tend to "over-call" DCIS and I will talk about some studies that showed this later. Some doctors tend to over-treat whereas others under-treat. The point is that nobody really knows, so it's important to get the facts and objective advice about your treatment options.

Most of our patients don't have a relapse, but working in a large referral center I see many patients whose DCIS has come back and I think, "If only the patient got the right treatment the first time." It's by understanding how, when, where, and why DCIS comes back that we can effectively treat *you* as an *individual* patient.

In fact, on the day I was writing this introduction, a patient was discussed at an MDT meeting I attended while in Europe who had a 20 mm "high-grade" DCIS treated by wide excision without radiation two years earlier. She now had a large recurrent area of DCIS with areas of invasive cancer. I strongly proposed that the risk of her cancer coming back was 30% without radiation with a 15% chance that the DCIS would come back as a real breast cancer. She is now facing a mastectomy and treatment to the lymph nodes and possible **chemotherapy** or **hormonal treatment**. As I will discuss later, this is a very real dilemma for women with DCIS. Some doctors are biased towards only surgical treatment, whereas others, including me, favor treatment with a lumpectomy and radiation or a mastectomy for most patients.

The reason I stress the word "individual" is that with DCIS of the breast it's not as simple as using a recipe-book approach. In one center I visited, the rule was that if DCIS was low-grade or if it was high-grade and less than about an inch or 25 mm, radiation wasn't necessary. I didn't quite agree with this and strongly advocate that you, the patient, understand the pros and cons of treatment and be actively involved in the decision-making process. It is not up to us as doctors to pick the "right" treatment for you, as there is no absolute right treatment. Some people are more prepared to take a risk than others and may forgo radiation treatment after a lumpectomy. Others, in my experience, want to reduce the risks as much as possible and prefer to add radiation or even have a mastectomy knowing that they have many years ahead of them and don't want to deal with any chance of a recurrence.

WHY ME?

There are many potential causes of DCIS, but the important things to note are:

- There may be some causes or aggravating factors of DCIS that you can change. For example, you can stop taking a birth control pill or HRT.

- There may be factors associated with your DCIS that you cannot change, for example, your family history or when you had your first child.

The best approach is not to be too hard on yourself. I see many patients who feel guilty because they wrongly perceive that their behavior may have caused their DCIS. Sometimes in life it depends on the roll of the dice and we can't really explain why something happens to us. Sometimes it may be for reasons that will take years to understand fully. It's important not to "rewind your tape"—to focus overly on the past or the guilt and regrets that might come with it—and not to "fast forward your tape"—to focus too much on the bewildering range of possibilities in the future. Rather, turn your energy toward the things that you can control.

Some factors that are usually quoted in books or women's magazines include:

- My period started early.

- I have always been overweight.

- I started the pill when I was sixteen.

- I took the pill for twenty years.

- I've taken hormone replacement therapy (HRT) for the last three years.

- My mother has had breast cancer.

- It's all the stress in my life.

- It's my job.

- It's the hormones they feed to chickens.

- It's the deodorant I've been using.

- It's the bra I've been wearing.

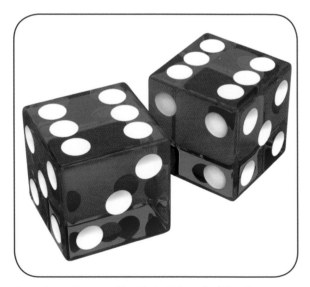

Sometimes it seems like it's just the roll of the dice.

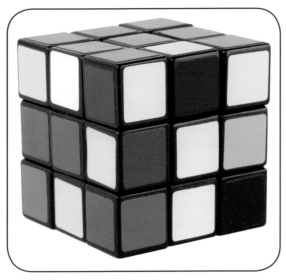

We really don't know exactly which factors cause DCIS.
(By permission of Seven Towns Ltd)

Quite frankly, it's not that simple. The development of DCIS is a complex Rubik's cube®. You may look in one direction and see all the blue bits lining up and one researcher may say that it's all genetic. You turn the cube around and another researcher states that it's all the hormones we've been using in Western society. You turn the cube around again and see that maybe it's something that you've been doing with your diet, the pill, or HRT.

Some studies have looked at risk factors for DCIS. One large study did show a link between taking HRT and DCIS. Another found a family history of breast cancer increased the risk of DCIS and one other found that the breast cancer gene carriers had an increased risk of DCIS of the higher grade variety (Kuerer et al. 2008).

Very few women with DCIS are thought to be linked in some way to alterations in the genes called **BRCA1 and BRCA2** (which is shorthand for breast cancer 1 and breast cancer 2). This is highest in families with a history of multiple members with breast cancer, where both breast and ovarian cancer are diagnosed in the same family, or in families with breast cancer diagnosed before the age of 50, or having an Eastern European (Ashkenazi) Jewish background. In a study of 369 women with DCIS tested for the BRCA1 or BRCA2 gene, mutations were found in three (0.8%) and 9 (2.4%) respectively (Claus et al. 2005). If your doctor suspects a genetic link, he or she may refer you and your family to a dedicated family history clinic and talk to you about arranging a blood test for the BRCA1 and BRCA2 gene changes or "mutations."

In summary, the dice have fallen in a particular way. You have DCIS, and really shouldn't dwell too much on what might have caused it. If you have been taking HRT, then yes, you should stop as it may have "fed" your cancer, particularly if your cancer is "hormone positive," or what we call "estrogen receptor (ER) positive."

Prior to the advent of breast screening, DCIS usually presented as a lump or a nipple discharge or rash. The nipple rash was called Paget's disease. I will talk about this later in "Control Point #8—What is Paget's Disease of the Nipple?"

DCIS is common in Western society, but not that common. Currently up to one in four abnormalities in the breast are DCIS and three in four are invasive breast cancers. It is partly because we are living longer and are now facing more and more chronic diseases such as heart disease, diabetes, and cancers of all types. Incidentally, most forms of DCIS have an exceptional **prognosis**, which approaches over 95% irrespective of how we treat you.

"DCIS" is not a great term. It is confused by the fact that the "C" stands for "carcinoma," which means cancer. Yes, it's a scary word, *but* it is a disease that can be beaten and most women are cured of DCIS. Others have argued that we should change the name to "DNIS" or ductal neoplasia in situ, but this recommendation hasn't really caught on.

I use the term "precancer" with my patients to stress that it's not "real" or invasive cancer as yet. It has not invaded the duct, in which case it would be called "invasive ductal carcinoma," but it remains *in situ*, a Latin term meaning "in place." For the rest of the book, I will call the condition DCIS.

UNDERSTANDING THE ANATOMY OF YOUR BREAST

I am not a gardener, but I find that most people have, at some time in their life, kept a garden or indoor plant or at least enjoyed walking through a public garden. My attempts at gardening have always been a total failure, mainly because I immerse myself in breast cancer and not gardening.

I do, however, find that examples from nature help you understand the many choices you'll face, and I will use them throughout the book. I like to call these points "Control Points" because they are a combination of important steps you need to take at the right time—important decisions and choices. This book will allow you to *take control* of these decisions by having the right information.

Before I give you the twenty essential "Control Points" you will need to navigate not only your new diagnosis but also an often complex health system, I will talk a little about how DCIS starts and what it looks like under a microscope. From there, I will give you the Control Points, which are either decision points where you will have to make a choice, or important points you need to think about to ensure that you get the best possible care.

The breast, believe it or not, is not unlike the Australian gum tree (Figure A). The trunk at the base of the plant is like the large ducts near the nipple. As we move toward the back of the breast and toward

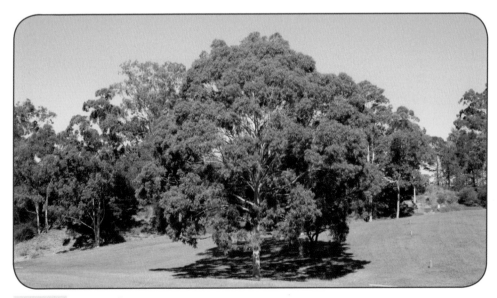

FIGURE A An Australian gum tree.

the skin, there are smaller and smaller branches and then smaller and smaller twigs. Where the twigs and the leaves meet, this is known as the **terminal duct lobular unit**. We've been told for years by various pathologists that this is where breast cancer actually begins. It is probably true in most cases. For some reason, the area where the leaf joins the twig becomes unstable and the cells can change.

Figure B shows a breast, the ducts (the small pipes that carry milk from the breast glands), and the breast glands (where the milk is produced during lactation). The leaves are the lobules where milk is produced, and the branches are the ducts.

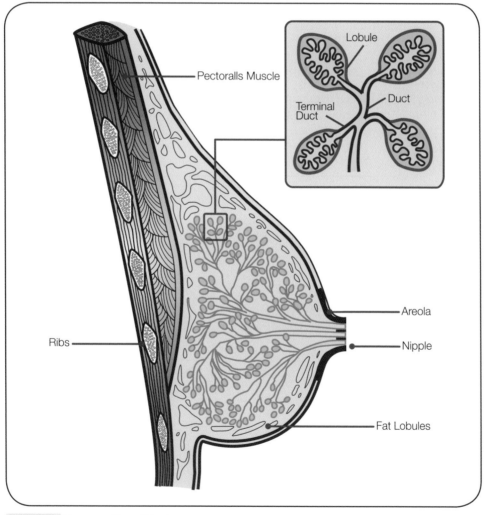

FIGURE B Cross-section of the breast.

James Going, a pathologist from Glascow in Scotland, published an elegant study of the duct system of the human breast (Going and Moffat 2004). He discovered that:

- the average breast has twenty-seven central ducts draining the breast

- the number of ducts ranged from eleven to forty-eight

- half of the breast was drained by only three ducts

- three-quarters of the breast was drained by the largest six ducts

- only seven ducts drained up and opened out to the skin of the nipple whereas the remainder were either just beneath it or tapered off away from the tip of the nipple

- there was overlapping of the duct systems (shown in Figure C).

Going's study showed that it is not always possible to access an abnormal duct system by probing the ducts visible at the tip of the nipple. He also postulated that the large differences in the size of DCIS between patients may simply be due to normal variation in the volume of the twenty-seven separate duct systems.

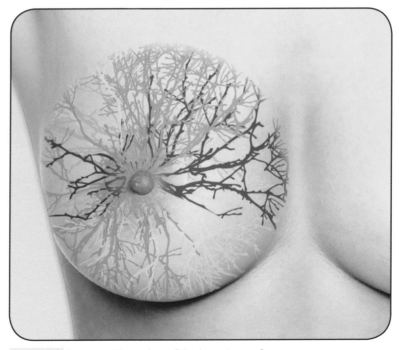

FIGURE C Ducts and branches of the breast seen face-on.

It is hard to know what makes the cells change. What you need to know is that if you obtain a little garden saw and cut through one of these ducts, you would normally see a hollow tube with a single lining of cells. Figure D shows what a branch or duct looks like when it is cut through.

With time, the cells can become heaped up. When the cells heap up a bit more, this is called hyperplasia, which means "too many cells." When the heaped-up cells don't look typical, this is called **atypia**, meaning not typical or not normal. These changes of hyperplasia or atypia are often present with DCIS and as I will show later can, at times, be difficult to distinguish from DCIS.

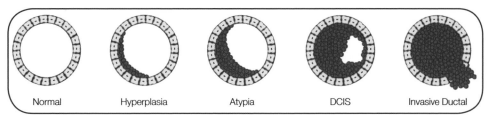

| Normal | Hyperplasia | Atypia | DCIS | Invasive Ductal |

FIGURE D Cross-section of a breast duct going from normal to invasive ductal carcinoma.

It's the second last diagram in Figure D that I really want you to concentrate on for now. If the cells begin to look like cancer cells and are still confined within the duct, it's called ductal carcinoma in situ, or DCIS. As mentioned, I call this "precancer" because the cells have not yet invaded through the duct, and I often explain this as a pipe that is very strong on the outside but contains some rust on the inside that has not yet penetrated the surface of the pipe. The real medical term is a "precancerous lesion" or "premalignant."

If you have been diagnosed with invasive carcinoma, the cancer has penetrated through the pipe—burst through the duct wall. This is also referred to as invasive ductal carcinoma or **infiltrating ductal carcinoma**, which means essentially the same thing—that there is an **invasive carcinoma** or you have a diagnosis of breast cancer.

If you have a large area of high-grade DCIS, there can sometimes be one or many tiny areas of invasion through the duct measuring up to 1 mm. This is often called microinvasion. DCIS is totally different to **lobular carcinoma in situ (LCIS)**, which is a type of change that starts in the "leaves" or **lobules** rather than the ducts. If you have LCIS, don't read any further as your doctor will explain to you that this is a marker of an increased risk of breast cancer in the future in either one of your breasts. LCIS will require close surveillance with regular mammograms and an **ultrasound**, sometimes tamoxifen or, after a lot of discussion, prophylactic removal of both of your breasts, particularly if you have a very strong family history of breast cancer (Visvanathan et al. 2013).

The lymphatic system is part of the immune system, which helps to fight infection and can stop cancer cells in the glands. DCIS, as a rule, does not spread to the lymph glands. Later I will discuss the role of sampling a gland in the armpit for selected patients with DCIS and show you that in some circumstances we do find some cells in the lymph gland, although this is very uncommon unless there are documented or suspected areas of microinvasion. If there are small areas of invasive cancer these cells can spread via small vessels, called lymphatics, that carry the fluid called lymph all around our body, including in the breast. Lymphatics, are connected to lymph glands or nodes, which are found in the armpit (also known as the axilla) and around the breastbone (the **sternum**) and collar bone (the clavicle).

Now that you've been told you have DCIS it is important to understand clearly what needs to be done. I'd like to go back to my garden example that I used in my first book, *Breast Cancer: Taking Control*. For patients who have breast cancer we talk about four garden patches.

The garden patches are like the four different **stages** in breast cancer (Figure E).

The first garden patch has a rose bush, and under this rose, there is a weed. Let's assume this weed is your breast cancer and the rose bush is your breast. This is called "stage 1."

The next garden patch looks okay, and there are no weeds in it. This next stage is like your "axilla" or armpit. If the weed or the cancer goes to this next garden patch, it is called "stage 2."

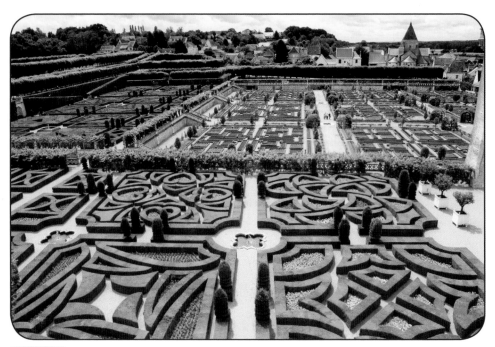

FIGURE E DCIS is like a seed from a weed that hasn't taken root in your garden.

A weed that spreads from under the rose bush to the next patch and the one after is like a large cancer that is very advanced in the breast and gland areas, which we call "stage 3."

A weed that affects a faraway part of the garden is like a cancer that affects different parts of the body, such as the liver or lungs, and is called "stage 4."

The good news about DCIS is that it hasn't even got to first base. The change is not even visible and it's often called "stage 0." It's a bit like a seed from a weed located in the patch of concrete at the center of the four garden patches of Figure E. It is close to being a "stage 1" cancer but hasn't even started to take root. It is still in situ or in-place and not a weed (or real cancer) as yet. So even though we talk about treating DCIS with similar treatments we use with real or invasive breast cancer, it's great that you have been diagnosed at such an early stage. Left alone, it is likely that your DCIS could have progressed to invasive cancer in a few years' time. It is likely to blow into the first garden patch, be fed, and potentially grow into a real cancer. But for now it's stage 0 and you have a great chance of being cured of DCIS and having a normal life expectancy.

However, it can be very confusing and the best thing to do right now is slow down, don't panic, and keep reading. It's only natural to be scared but having the right information at your fingertips will help you take control.

Ruth's Story

Towards the end of 1993 I was working in an office when one of the staff told me she had booked the women in our office to go for a breast screen in a van parked in the shopping center. She told me "There is one in every group and the van is air conditioned so it will be lovely to go to a cool place to be in those machines." At the time I was 41 and like many women, was dismissive of any need for me to be screened. There is no history in my family, I breast-fed all my children and besides, I was too young!

After the scan, I was recalled to the assessment clinic and having big breasts I thought the staff at Penrith had not got them properly in the machines, so didn't take my husband or any support person with me. However, as the afternoon wore on with the concentration of attention, that is, mammogram, ultrasound and biopsy all on my left breast, I knew things were looking serious.

I was not surprised when at 5.30 pm I was called into what looked like a panel of medical staff and was given the news that I needed to see a surgeon with regard to what looked like lines of calcifications (DCIS) on the inside milk ducts of my left breast. In trying to make light of the situation I told the panel that may be happening to my left breast but I had won tickets to *The Gondoliers* at the Sydney Opera House for that evening and I would deal with my breast the next day. I rang my husband and let him know before I left the clinic. On arrival home my then 10-year-old daughter asked why I was upset, but given the babysitter was expected I told her that I would talk to her the next day. I did see a surgeon the next day and was told that I could have a partial mastectomy or a mastectomy. I was told that my nipple would not need to be touched. Being only 41 I was not ready for a mastectomy (and my left breast was my and my husband's favorite!) so I elected for a partial mastectomy. We did explain to our children who were 10, 9 and 7 what was happening and tried not to alarm them.

Quite wide margins were taken. The part I enjoyed least was having all the needles/ wires placed in my breast, standing and being still prior to the operation. I also found it difficult that my own mother felt she would "catch" the disease and was not able to be supportive. This opened up a lot of issues for me around mothering, my relationship with my mother and the nurturing part of my body which was affected. Subsequently I sought counseling support.

A fond memory I have is of one of my children lying on top of me and kissing my scars better. I of course have always "kissed" the kids' scars better. Whilst I was told I may need to have a series of operations if the DCIS recurred, it is now twenty years on and the DCIS has never returned. I continue to have annual checkups.

Joan's Story

I was seventy years old when I went for my routine breast screen mammogram. I was recalled to an Assessment Clinic and had additional tests including a core biopsy. The staff at the clinic asked me if I wanted to come back the following week to the clinic or to see my general practitioner to obtain the results.

As I was working I thought I would drop in and see my general practitioner a week later after work. My GP asked, "How are you?" and I said, "You know better than me." He then immediately said, "You've got cancer." I nearly fell off my chair and was in tears.

Later that evening my daughter did some research for me on the Internet and discovered DCIS was not cancer at all but a type of precancer. I still get teary when I think of that day and realize now that I should have taken somebody with me.

My GP was excellent in referring me quickly to a breast surgeon but I am still thinking of changing doctors because of the way he handled me at this very emotional time.

PART 1

"SHOCK CONTROL"

TAKING CONTROL IMMEDIATELY AFTER DIAGNOSIS

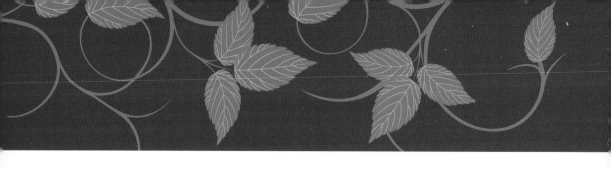

CONTROL POINT #1

WHAT ON EARTH IS "DCIS"?

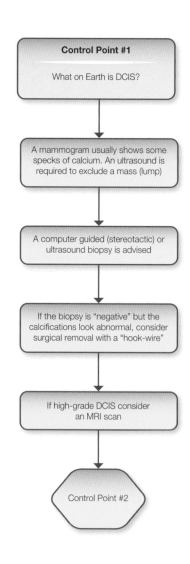

Control Point #1

What on Earth is DCIS?

A mammogram usually shows some specks of calcium. An ultrasound is required to exclude a mass (lump)

A computer guided (stereotactic) or ultrasound biopsy is advised

If the biopsy is "negative" but the calcifications look abnormal, consider surgical removal with a "hook-wire"

If high-grade DCIS consider an MRI scan

Control Point #2

It Pays to Understand What DCIS Really Means

When you look back at the incidence of DCIS for women over 50, there was a rapid increase in the diagnosis of DCIS in the United States beginning around 1983, and once again in the late 80s as mammography use become more widespread (Figure 1.1). The incidence of DCIS started to go down again after 2001. I'll explain my theory in a moment. For every 100,000 women in their 50s, almost ninety will be diagnosed with DCIS each and every year.

In these early years, though, DCIS was basically classed as **comedo** or **non-comedo** based simply on its architectural appearance (Figures 1.2–1.5). I am including this older classification in this book as I still do see reports from time to time using this term. For a variety of reasons that are not that important, the early pathologists called DCIS which had a large area of dead cells in the center with calcium (as in Figure 1.3) "comedo" and the remainder (Figures 1.2, 1.4, 1.5) "non-comedo."

Basically, as shown in the introduction in Figure D, the darker cells in the center of the DCIS are cells that have outgrown their blood supply and died off from lack of food. Normally, there is a tiny blood vessel that supplies oxygen and nutrients to the single layer of cells lining your ducts, as with the duct labeled "Normal" in Figure D. When the abnormal cells pile up on each other, the cells in the center starve. It's a bit like your teenage son inviting ten of his friends over and raiding your fridge for food. Some of them have to starve. When cells are starved of oxygen, they actually die. In medicine, this is called "**necrosis**." When a cell dies in the body, one healing mechanism is for the body to calcify it. This is one of the main reasons we see calcium specks on your mammogram. Because some of the cells still get oxygen, they don't die or calcify and may not be seen on your mammogram. Sometimes your DCIS may produce some secretions, which then calcify. Later, I will explain the different types of calcification that may be present in your breast X-ray or mammogram.

The problem with incidence rates is that how pathologists defined DCIS has changed over time, and many of the older cancer registries have not moved to newer classifications. Hence, classifications as "comedo" versus "non-comedo" are of interest, but really won't help all that much in terms of treatment.

So if we go back to the U.S. incidence data, you can see in Figure 1.1 certain important changes over time. In the 1980s, there were some key papers published by the masters of pathology, Paul Peter Rosen, David Page, and Edwin Fisher, who started guiding pathologists about how to differentiate the steps before DCIS (as shown in Figure D). This differentiation included hyperplasia (where the cells inside the duct in Figure D are beginning to replicate and pile up on each other), or atypical hyperplasia (where the cells are beginning to look unusual or "not typical" from DCIS). I suspect that a large part of the increase in rates of DCIS from 1980 to 1985 was partly a change in the threshold that an individual pathologist used to differentiate hyperplasia from DCIS, and partly because of

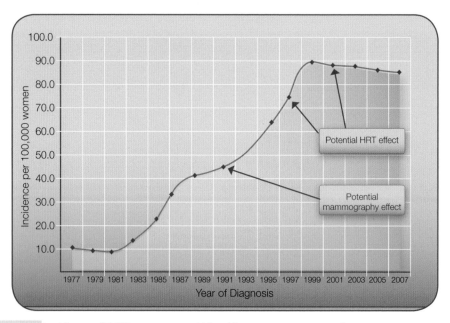

Figure 1.1 Incidence of DCIS per 100,000 U.S. white women 50 years of age or over.

the increasing use of mammography in that time period. Mammography use was very patchy at the time—the equipment was very basic and the images of poor quality. The use of mammography began to really take off in the late 80s when the rate of comedo DCIS began to increase.

The rate of comedo DCIS, however, then stabilized and has not gone up since 1991. Of note, however, the rate of the lower-grade non-comedo DCIS went up again in 1990 and continued to increase until 2001, probably due to the increasing use of hormone replacement therapy (HRT) at that time (Reeves et al. 2006). After the so-called "HRT scare" of 2001 and 2002 where two studies publicized widely in the media showed a strong link between taking HRT and breast cancer, its use halved in many countries, and this reduced the incidence of DCIS (and invasive cancer) as shown by the decreasing incidence from 2001 to 2007 (Figure 1.1). Luo et al. (2013) also found some evidence linking the increased incidence of DCIS with HRT.

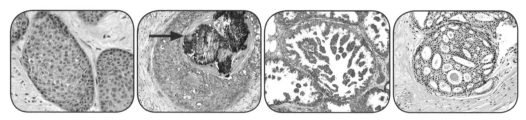

Figure 1.2 DCIS with "solid" architecture as seen under a microscope **Figure 1.3** DCIS with "comedo" architecture with central calcium spots (arrowed) **Figure 1.4** Micro-papillary DCIS **Figure 1.5** DCIS with "cribriform" architecture like a "lace tablecloth".

How Common Is DCIS?

It can be difficult to estimate the number of women (and the few men) who are diagnosed with DCIS each year. Because it is not yet cancer, many registries have not been collecting this data.

In the U.S., it was estimated that about 62,000 women were diagnosed with DCIS in 2009 (Jemal et al. 2009), compared to 192,000 women with invasive breast cancer. That is, about one in four significant breast problems are DCIS. These figures are assumptions based on data collection from a few cancer registries. Perhaps more accurate data is available from Australia, where about 7% of all cases of significant breast disease (invasive cancer or DCIS) were DCIS in 1993, rising to 11.3% in 2005. It has been estimated by the Australian Institute of Health and Welfare that there were 13,600 women with invasive breast cancer in 2009, and therefore a total of about 1,700 women with DCIS. So if you are in Australia, it is estimated that four women like yourself are diagnosed with DCIS every single day.

In the U.K., it has been estimated that 45,700 women were diagnosed with invasive cancer in 2007 (Cancer Research UK 2010). I have estimated that about 5,800 women are diagnosed with this disease every year, or over fifteen women every single day in the U.K.

I am boring you with all these statistics just to let you know that you are not alone and that many thousands of women struggle with the diagnosis of DCIS every year. And most women beat DCIS and avoid a future diagnosis of breast cancer.

How Is DCIS Diagnosed?

It is highly likely that your DCIS was detected by an abnormality on your mammogram. Occasionally, it is picked up by accident after a surgeon removes something else from your breast that turns out to be harmless, like a benign fibrous growth. Sometimes, a small lump may be discovered. Some patients are diagnosed with Paget's disease, which is DCIS involving the ducts behind the nipple and can progress to involve the tip of the nipple and even the skin of the **areola**. (I'll talk more about Paget's disease in "Control Point #8 – What Is Paget's Disease of the Nipple?") At other times, DCIS may be diagnosed after blood is seen coming out of the nipple.

Assuming you have had an area of **microcalcification** in the breast picked up on your mammogram (Figure 1.6), this area would have special X-rays called **magnification views** (Figure 1.7), where the abnormal area is magnified so the radiologist can more easily see the abnormal area of calcifications. You or your doctor cannot feel microcalcifications. The calcifications

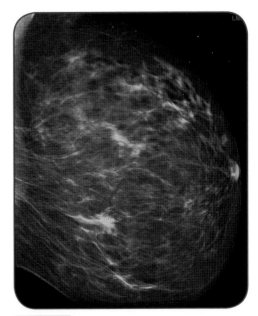

Figure 1.6 DCIS (arrowed) first detected by a standard mammogram.

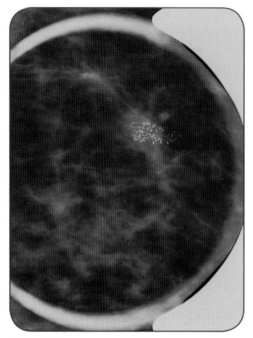

occur in four ways: (1) in groups, known as "clusters," which can vary in size or shape; (2) in grouped straight lines, known as "linear," inside the breast duct; (3) in branched-out patterns, known as "branching," into two or more ducts; or (4) in casting-type patterns, known as "casting," on the inside of the breast ducts. Calcifications that are more circular than straight are called "granular." All these types of calcifications are considered to be suspicious and always need a **biopsy**.

Calcifications are particularly suspicious if they occur in one part or segment of the duct system. By now you may have had a **core biopsy** where a small sample of the breast and the calcifications are taken using a thick needle. It's a bit like a farmer taking core samples of the soil on his farm. You would have had your breast "fixed" in position using the plates on a mammogram machine. Sometimes the core biopsy is done with your breast placed in a hole on a specially made bed called a **prone table** (Figure 1.8) or using upright procedures using a specially modified mammogram machine (Figure 1.9). Once the core biopsy has been done, always check that the radiologist has X-rayed the core samples to make sure any calcium spots seen

Figure 1.7 "Magnification views" show calcium to be of coarse granular variety and suspicious of DCIS.

on your original mammogram have been adequately sampled by being seen on an X-ray of the cores (Figure 1.10). Sometimes if there is a suggestion of some thickening or haziness on your mammogram,

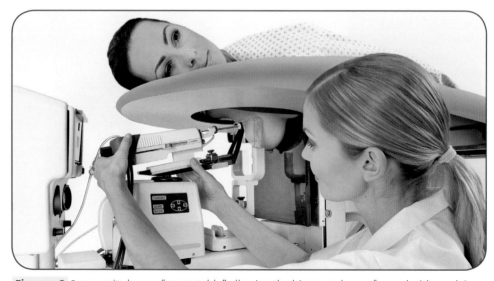

Figure 1.8 Some units have a "prone table" allowing the biopsy to be performed with you lying on your front with your breast accessible below via a hole in the bed.

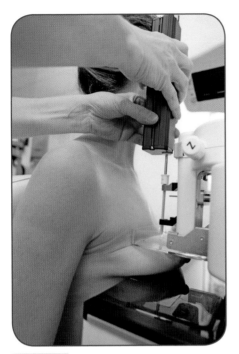

Figure 1.9 A core biopsy is done with a special device attached to the mammogram machine with you in the upright position.

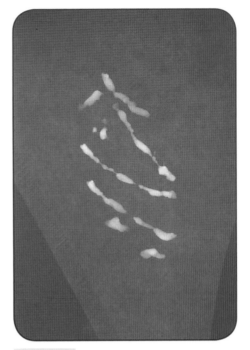

Figure 1.10 X-rays are done after the core biopsies are taken to ensure that calcium is visible confirming the right spot has been sampled.

an ultrasound is also done over the calcification. If the area of your microcalcification was very small, radiologists these days normally put in a clip that can be seen on a subsequent mammogram (see Figure 1.11). Sometimes the core biopsy procedure removes all the calcification making it extremely difficult for the surgeon to know what area to remove. The clip is also useful if something doesn't quite add up and your doctors need to "retrace their steps" trying to find where the abnormal area was located in your original mammogram and what area was actually biopsied if, for example, the final pathology came back unexpectedly benign when DCIS was highly suspected.

Since the late 1990s, more and more research has been done comparing the use of breast **magnetic resonance imaging (MRI)** scans to that of

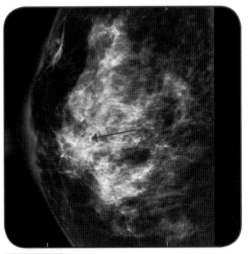

Figure 1.11 Core biopsies can remove all the calcification so sometimes a small, non-magnetic titanium clip is placed where the abnormal calcium was located (arrow).

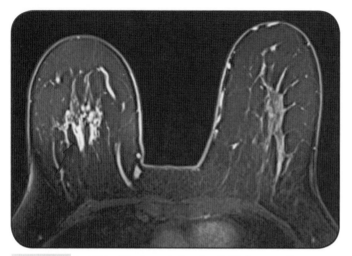

Figure 1.12 An MRI of the breast showing DCIS (arrowed).

mammography (Figure 1.12). An MRI does not use radiation (X-rays) but a strong magnet and radio waves. It involves an injection called gadolinium given through an intravenous line. This is often taken up by the DCIS or a hidden cancer, which can then alert the radiologist of a problem. You will lie on your front with your breasts hanging down into cushioned openings. Before the test, tell your health care provider if you have any metal parts in your body (brain aneurysm clips, heart valves, pacemakers, cochlear implants, artificial joints, vascular stents) which could be affected by the strong magnet. The gadolinium contrast dye is also contraindicated if you have significant kidney disease.

The MRI scanner is shaped like a tunnel and some patients find it a little claustrophobic (also see Figure 15.1). During the MRI, the person who operates the machine will watch you (and can also hear you) through a glass screen. The machine makes a fair bit of noise and earmuffs are worn during the test. The test takes between thirty and sixty minutes. An MRI is not a replacement for mammography and ultrasound.

In September 2009, the National Cancer Institute (NCI) and the Office of Medical Applications of Research of the National Institutes of Health held a conference to explore and assess the current scientific knowledge regarding the diagnosis and management of DCIS. They found that:

- MRI is more sensitive than mammography for detecting DCIS in more than one part of the breast known as **multicentric disease**.

- The results of studies comparing MRI with mammography and the final pathology size of your DCIS are inconsistent. Overall, MRI is believed to slightly improve on mammography but has been found to both underestimate and overestimate the size of your DCIS.

- MRI used to detect **occult DCIS** (meaning DCIS which is hidden or not seen on your mammogram and ultrasound) or breast cancer in the opposite breast, can produce **false-positive** and **false-negative** results.

In the NCI review of this and several other controversial areas, evidence was documented which extended to over 500 pages. The report concluded that an:

- MRI detected additional areas of unsuspected disease in other parts of the breast in only 6 out of 100 scans.

- MRI overestimated the size of the DCIS compared to the final pathology size for one in five patients and also underestimated it in one in five patients.

- MRI found a breast cancer in the opposite breast in 6 of 100 patients.

The 31-page consumer statement, which is certainly more digestible for you as a patient, can be downloaded from http://consensus.nih.gov/2009/dcisstatement.htm. If you are a student or doctor, the full evidence can be found at http://consensus.nih.gov/2009/dcis.htm.

At this stage, I am not routinely recommending MRI scans for my patients but will consider it for patients with a strong family history, younger patients whose breasts are quite dense with a core biopsy diagnosed area of DCIS, patients with high grade DCIS, those few patients who present with a lump which is DCIS, patients with Paget's disease and potentially for patients with large areas of DCIS where there is some concern about its true extent with mammography. Certainly, in Australia and the U.K., there is no government funding or rebates for MRI in this setting and the cost is several hundreds of dollars.

Most of the time, as DCIS cannot be felt, a procedure called "wire localization" will be performed by a radiologist on the night before or the morning of your surgery (Figure 1.13). This involves inserting a guide wire (called a "**hookwire**") via X-ray or, less frequently, ultrasound control and positioning it just beyond the abnormal area in your mammogram. When you're under anesthetic, the surgeon will follow the wire to find and remove the DCIS (where the tip of the wire, or the "hook," is), along with a rim of surrounding healthy tissue, and then remove the wire with the piece of breast tissue attached. If the area is quite large or if there are two areas, sometimes two wires are inserted at either end of the calcium spots. This is called "bracketing" of the abnormal area. Once removed, the tissue is X-rayed to make sure the calcium spots don't reach the outside edge of the specimen. This is called a **specimen X-ray** or specimen radiograph. Many surgeons wait to look at the X-ray and then make a decision whether or not to take an extra "shave" if the edge is close to the calcium spots; whereas others believe that it is better to look at the X-ray when they have the final pathology report available rather than prolonging your time under anesthetic or potentially removing more healthy tissue unnecessarily (Figure 1.14).

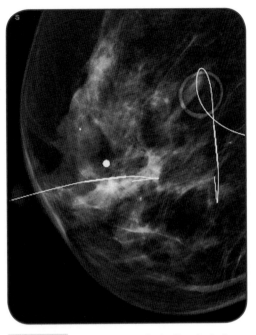

Figure 1.13 A guide wire called a "hookwire" is inserted before surgery in the radiology department to guide the surgeon to the area of calcification.

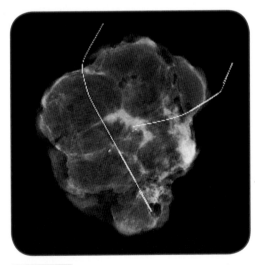

Figure 1.14 Generally while you are still under the anesthetic, the excised area of your breast is also X-rayed to check that the surgeon has gotten the calcified area with normal-appearing surrounding tissue.

A not uncommon situation is when you are diagnosed as having hyperplasia after an initial core biopsy (one of the steps before DCIS shown in Figure D, page 11), but when the abnormal area is removed by the surgeon, the final pathology actually shows DCIS. Another situation that can happen from time to time is that after the initial core biopsy is called "DCIS" the abnormal area removed by the surgeon does not show DCIS at all. Table 1.1 below shows one large study that studied this question very carefully. In this large multicenter study from Holland, 858 women had a core biopsy using very accurate guidance called a **stereotactic biopsy**. The study was called the COBRA study (COre Biopsy after RAdiological localisation). A digital mammogram was used and at least five cores were taken of each abnormality on the mammogram. All discrepancies between the core biopsy and the final surgical specimen were reviewed by a panel of five doctors. So, in other words, this was a very careful, well-conducted study (Verkooijen 2002).

Table 1.1 Comparison of a core biopsy using a local anesthetic with removal (surgical biopsy) of the abnormal area on a mammogram

SURGICAL BIOPSY					
Core Biopsy	Total	% DCIS	% Invasive	% High-Risk	% Normal or Benign
Normal or Benign	352	5%	1%	4%	91%
High-Risk	26	19%	4%	39%	39%
DCIS	190	75%	17%	3%	5%
Invasive	290	1%	98%	0%	1%
Total	858	20%	37%	3%	40%

Firstly, when a core biopsy showed DCIS, then in three out of four patients (75%), DCIS was confirmed as the final pathology following a surgical biopsy where the abnormal area in the breast was removed using a general anesthetic. However in 17% of cases, there was actually a real (invasive) cancer there. If this has happened to you, the rest of this book is not relevant and you should be reading my other book, *Breast Cancer: Taking Control.*

If your core biopsy showed DCIS and the surgical biopsy showed what the investigators called a high-risk lesion (3% chance) or was "normal or benign" (5% chance), then your original core biopsy will have to be reviewed very, very carefully. High-risk abnormalities in this study were defined as hyperplasia (see Figure D) or LCIS. This only happened in a handful of patients but the dilemma here is whether or not your original core biopsy was an "overcall" and really could be categorized as hyperplasia where close monitoring with regular mammograms is all that would be required, or whether indeed you did have DCIS and it was all totally cored out during the original procedure.

What your doctor is trying to work out is if your original core biopsy was a "true positive" and it really was DCIS, or a "false positive" and really should have been classified, in retrospect, as hyperplasia or indeed a benign lesion. Sometimes the original core biopsy sample may be sent for a second opinion from another pathologist.

You may have faced another frustrating situation in which your core biopsy was a false negative. Your mammographic abnormality was obviously of some concern, but the core biopsy was "normal" or "benign." Your doctors then recommended surgical removal and it did in fact show DCIS (5% risk in this study) or invasive cancer (1%). The good news here is that your doctors persisted in getting to the bottom of the abnormality on your mammogram and finally worked out what was going on.

Can My Diagnosis of DCIS Be Wrong?

It is unlikely that your diagnosis of DCIS is incorrect. However, it always pays to ask questions. In one famous study, a pathologist sent around ten pathology slides of ductal lesions including DCIS, hyperplasia, or atypia to five of the U.S.A.'s most highly respected, experienced, and well-published pathologists at the time. The results are shown in Table 1.2. As you can see, it was a bit all over the place. There was not a single ductal type lesion for which all pathologists agreed upon the diagnosis, and if your case was sent to pathologist "P1" you were more likely to be diagnosed with DCIS whereas "P5" didn't diagnose DCIS for any case (Rosai 1991).

There a few "buts" here though. All the lesions were very difficult to diagnose and tended at the lower-grade end of the spectrum, and there were no cases of the easier to diagnose comedo-type DCIS. This is always a little harder to diagnose than high-grade or "comedo" DCIS. The pathologists were not given any real guidelines. Further, they were only given a single slide sample of each case. In reality, when a pathologist looks at your case of DCIS, he or she may be looking at up to 100 slides. In short, what I am saying is that this study in Table 1.2 is not real life. In another study from New Hampshire,

Table 1.2 A study showing how five expert pathologists can disagree with each other when reviewing the same ten difficult cases of possible DCIS

		PATHOLOGIST				
		1	2	3	4	5
	1	AH	AH	AH	H	H
	2	AH	AH	N	H	H
	3	DCIS	DCIS	AH	DCIS	AH
	4	DCIS	AH	DCIS	H	AH
Case	5	AH	AH	H	H	H
Number	6	DCIS	ALH	DCIS	AH	H
	7	AH	H	AH	H	H
	8	AH	H	H	H	H
	9	AH	AH	AH	AH	H
	10	DCIS	AH	H	H	H

H= Hyperplasia; **AH**= Atypical hyperplasia; **ALH**=Atypical lobular hyperplasia; **DCIS**=Ductal carcinoma in situ

community pathologists rather than expert breast pathologists were asked to describe forty cases of DCIS using three international DCIS classifications.

In contrast to Rosai's study, closer correlations were found between the community pathologists and the three experts after they were given written guidelines about each classification (Wells et al. 2000) confirming the importance of written guidelines reported by Schnitt et al. (1992). Nevertheless, I have had several patients sent to me over the years with very small areas of low-grade DCIS (under 5 mm) where a second opinion has shown it to be normal or just hyperplasia.

If there is some doubt, ask your surgeon to inquire about sending your slides off for a second opinion. In my experience, high-grade DCIS is hardly ever misdiagnosed as it has a far more predictable pattern under the microscope and hardly ever needs a second opinion. The only special situation is if you have been diagnosed with DCIS after previous radiation to the breast. The breast undergoes significant changes and sometimes these changes may even mimic DCIS.

Is DCIS Overdiagnosed?

The short answer is probably yes. As mentioned above, the diagnosis of DCIS is not black or white. There is a lot of gray in the middle and, as Rosai's study found, some pathologists are more inclined to call a "borderline" breast lesion DCIS, whereas others have a higher threshold and are more likely to call it "hyperplasia" or "atypia" (see Figure D, page 11).

Overdiagnosing DCIS is not a new phenomenon. Probably the first doctor to define DCIS was in fact the professor of surgery from Harvard University in Boston, Dr J. Collins Warren (Warren 1907). In his publication he states:

> To the lay mind a tumor of the breast is so suggestive of cancer that the patient is quite ready to submit to any measure, however radical, for its relief. Uncertainty as to the true nature of cysts of the breast has given rise in the professional mind to a diversity of opinions. By one a cyst is considered a harmless lesion which may be let alone, and this advice is often given, as the physician fears to place the patient in the hands of a surgeon who is inclined to amputate, as a routine treatment, every breast, whether it be the seat of cyst or a malignant growth.

In this classic publication, he first describes a build-up of cells in the duct, which is normally lined with only one cell and cautions against overdiagnosis and overtreatment. One hundred years later, we still face many of the same dilemmas!

There has been extensive debate about overdiagnosis of DCIS and invasive cancer with screening. Could the DCIS have remained dormant in your lifetime? Maybe. Could the treatment cause more harm than good? Maybe.

In one of the first trials showing a benefit from screening from Sweden, the overdiagnosis rate was estimated to be less than 5%; whereas in a modeling study from Australia, it was estimated to be up to 42% (Duffy et al. 2005 and Morrell et al. 2010). The truth is probably somewhere in between and probably on the lower side, but the reality is that this sort of debate really doesn't help you when you have been told that you have DCIS. Leave this sort of debate to the statisticians and epidemiologists. For now, we have to work out how to treat you.

You have now been told you have DCIS. No matter what the news headlines say about overdiagnosis, with certain quarters claiming that breast screening doesn't work because it overdiagnoses DCIS, the point is that many of these studies have been written by statisticians who have never examined a patient nor had to describe what DCIS really is; nor have they seen patients who progressed when DCIS was not treated properly in the first place.

Understanding Your Type of DCIS

The definition of DCIS has changed over the years as pathologists have used more sophisticated techniques with increasingly powerful microscopes and special stains and genetics tests on the breast tissue that is removed. To be frank, I am not sure if anyone totally understands the true complexity of DCIS. Pathologists have struggled with various classifications over the years, and I'll mention a few of the most important ones below as it may vary from treatment center to treatment center.

Over time (particularly in the late 80s and early 90s when there was a substantial increase in the number of women diagnosed with DCIS due to the start of breast-screening programs), pathologists starting classifying DCIS into the comedo or non-comedo subtype. As I was researching this book, I noticed that many women on various Web sites were still talk about "comedo" DCIS and many were asking what it really means. So this term is still out there being used today.

The earliest reference I can find about this was from Bloodgood (1908) where he mentions the term "comedo adenocarcinoma" and describes it as the "least malignant form of cancer of the breast." He describes himself and the "father of mastectomy," William Halstead, operating together on such a patient and when they squeezed the removed abnormal breast tissue, he stated that: "worm-like comedo bodies can be expressed. The appearance of this tumor is absolutely characteristic—once seen it will never be forgotten."

So basically, all that "necrotic" or "dead" material in the center of the duct can actually be squeezed like a facial pimple or acne.

The most common types of DCIS are of four main patterns or "architectural types":

- Solid DCIS—here the DCIS fills the whole duct without necrosis or calcification in the center (Figure 1.2).
- Comedo DCIS—this is when the cells in the center of the solid type of DCIS die off (necrosis) and calcify (Figure 1.3).
- Papillary/Micropapillary DCIS—these tumors have multiple fronds or finger-like projections. These eventually fuse together forming a "Roman arch" type appearance (Figure 1.4).
- Cribriform DCIS—the cells here form a "lace tablecloth" type appearance (Figure 1.5).

In "Control Point #13 – What Does My Pathology Report Really Mean?," I will go into more detail about the sort of changes the pathologist is looking for and will be talking about important aspects that may affect how you are treated. This will include: your "**margins**" of how much normal breast tissue there is between your surgeon's edge of resection and the DCIS, the grade of the DCIS, and the presence or absence of necrosis and calcification.

We still don't really understand how your DCIS has developed. For example, it is widely believed that atypical ductal hyperplasia (ADH) shown in Figure D on page 11 progresses sometimes, but not always, to low-grade DCIS but not high-grade or comedo DCIS. It was thought that low-grade and high-grade DCIS have different pathways of evolution or development but not everyone agrees. In one study of 200 DCIS tumors it was not unusual for the one type of DCIS to have areas ranging from low- to intermediate- to high-grade areas. Nearly half of the cases had different grades of tumor in different areas. The authors also found different types of genetic signatures on various types of DCIS, and they even suggested that many patients with low-grade DCIS may with time progress to high-grade DCIS and then to invasive cancer (Allred et al. 2008). So, in effect, what I am saying is that this categorization into low- or high-grade DCIS may be a figment of our imagination and, biologically, they may all be interrelated.

What Does My Mammogram Tell Me about My DCIS?

Mammography is one of the most important tests in determining what needs to be done to remove DCIS. Several studies have tried to correlate the appearance on your mammogram with the ultimate diagnosis. As mentioned earlier, DCIS usually, but not always, appears as areas of very fine calcifications called "microcalcifications" and usually the area is magnified so the doctor who reads the mammogram, a radiologist, can better evaluate their size, shape, and distribution (Figure 1.6). Occasionally, DCIS may present as a small lump or "mass," which may or may not be visible on the mammogram but may often be seen by an ultrasound. In one large study of 909 patients treated in Bordeaux, France, between 1980 and 1999, DCIS presented in the following ways:

- Abnormal mammogram: 76%
- Nipple Discharge: 12%
- Lump: 12%.

Of the 108 women with a nipple discharge, 96 were bloody or **serous** (Barreau et al. 2005). **Serous fluid** is clear and slightly yellow. It's the type of fluid found in a blister formed on your feet after wearing very tight, new shoes.

In a similar study conducted to see how DCIS presented over time, Tunon-de-Lara et al. (2001) found that before 1980, 58% of patients with DCIS had a nipple discharge and 44% had a lump; whereas since 1990, only 8% had nipple discharge and 13% had a lump. Since 1990, most women have had an abnormal mammogram, with 84% having microcalcification.

In an Australian study, about 80 to 85% of 335 women aged over 50 presented with an abnormal mammogram compared to about 50% of the 83 women aged under 50 at the time of diagnosis who normally presented with a lump (Shugg et al. 2002).

This is some of what we know so far about some of the differences between high and low-grade DCIS:

- High-grade DCIS is nearly always calcified (nine out of ten patients) whereas low-grade DCIS is only calcified in five out of ten cases, making it more difficult to diagnose and follow up.

- The calcium in high-grade DCIS seems to be indicative of the final dimension of the DCIS and is more likely to be "**casting**" or "**linear**" or "**branching**" (Figure 1.15) or coarse "**granular**" (Figure 1.7). The calcium in low-grade DCIS is more likely to be coarse granular (Figure 1.7) or fine granular (powdery) and not represent the full extent of the DCIS (Figure 1.16).

- High-grade DCIS is more likely than low-grade DCIS to spread behind the nipple, and special magnification X-rays of the mammogram behind the nipple may detect some calcium in that area.

- An MRI scan of the breast is better in showing high-grade DCIS than low-grade DCIS (Figure 1.12).

Table 1.3 shows the results of a well-conducted study correlating the grade of the DCIS and the preoperative abnormality found on the mammogram. Significantly, high-grade DCIS was nearly always associated with microcalcification, which was usually located in one segment of the breast, and had a linear or coarse granular pattern. Low-grade DCIS was associated with microcalcification in only half of the patients and tended to be granular rather than linear and in clusters rather than in a segment of the breast (De Roos et al. 2004).

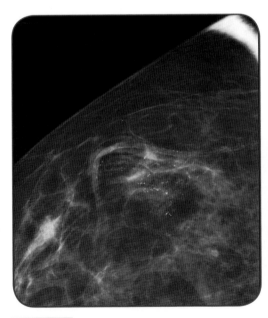

Figure 1.15 Linear and casting type calcification consistent with high-grade DCIS.

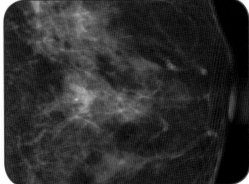

Figure 1.16 Fine granular or powdery calcification consistent with low-grade DCIS.

Table 1.3 Correlation between grade and mammographic appearance of DCIS

	GRADE		
Microcalcifications	Low (17%)	Intermediate (45%)	High (38%)
Present			
Yes	53%	73%	89%
No	47%	37%	11%
Distribution			
Segmental	20%	39%	51%
Clustered	80%	61%	49%
Pattern			
Linear ("casting")	20%	13%	67%
Coarse granular	80%	84%	82%
Fine granular	50%	39%	18%

Adapted from de Roos et al. (2004)

What Happens if DCIS Is Left Untreated?

The early studies of DCIS basically left DCIS untreated or treated only with a lumpectomy. One of the first studies of untreated DCIS was the original description by Sir James Paget (1874). While on sabbatical in Oxford in 2010, I managed to retrieve Paget's original paper from the archives of the Bodlean Library whilst researching this book. Paget wrote the following when talking about DCIS of the nipple:

> . . . But it has happened that in every case which I have been able to watch, cancer of the mammary gland has followed within at the most two years, and usually within one year.

This is perhaps one of the earliest descriptions of the progression of DCIS if left untreated. I will be writing further about DCIS involving the nipple in "Control Point #8 – What Is Paget's Disease of the Nipple?" Another study by a pathologist named David Page reviewed a very large series of "benign" biopsies from 29 patients. After careful reevaluation, the "benign" biopsies were reclassified as low-grade DCIS (Sanders 2005). What this study found was that eleven patients (38%) developed invasive (or real) breast cancer usually within ten years after their diagnosis and five patients (17%) died of breast cancer.

There is a tendency in some treatment centers to consider low-grade or non-comedo DCIS as benign but left untreated without good surgical margins, radiotherapy, or mastectomy, it may come back and cause problems. For this reason and based on some other studies that I will show in "Control Point #16 – Do I Need Radiation Therapy?," the evidence suggests that DCIS is a forerunner or a precursor to invasive cancer and needs to be discussed with you prior to treatment.

This is the obvious dilemma. If we leave your DCIS totally alone after a lumpectomy, it sometimes, but not always, progresses to real cancer; whereas if we treat you with a mastectomy or a lumpectomy and radiation, you will have to put up with side effects. In "Control Point #14 – What Is My Prognosis?," I will try to tease out how high the risks are of a recurrence of DCIS or an invasive cancer based on the size of your DCIS, its grade, and other factors such as the extent of surgery or your margins.

Defining the "Dilemmas of DCIS"

As you can see from the detail above, there are many dilemmas surrounding DCIS that will at first make you feel you are in some sort of roller coaster ride. Sometimes there is no right answer so be patient with your health-care team as they try to disentangle an often very complex situation where the X-ray picture may not be totally in step with the final pathology report. Some examples of dilemmas are the following:

- Is the abnormality DCIS or could it really be atypia or hyperplasia? (Figure D)
- What is the overall size of the DCIS, and what is the correlation between the size of the abnormal area as compared to the size of the final pathology?
- Why is it that although the DCIS may have been picked up early your doctors are recommending a mastectomy?
- Is breast screening overdiagnosing DCIS?
- What is the optimal use of radiation?
- How do I explain DCIS to my friends?

And so on and so on . . .

In the following chapters, I'll try my best to bring you up to date with the latest information to help you take control of some or all of these dilemmas. In "Control Point #2 – How Do I Find the Right Treatment Team?," I will firstly touch on some of the real communication issues which can occur between you and your doctors and then how to convey some or all of the information you receive to members of your family, friends, and colleagues.

CONTROL POINT #1 – WHAT ON EARTH IS "DCIS"?

WARNING Rushing into treatment for DCIS is unnecessary. You have plenty of time to get information and make an informed decision.

TIP If you are diagnosed with a very small "low-grade" DCIS measuring less than 5 mm, it may pay to ask for a second opinion from a specialist in breast pathology.

REMEMBER Understand that your breast condition has been picked up early before it has become a "real" or invasive breast disease, and you have an exceptionally high cure rate of close to 99 to 100%.

Julienne's Story

About five years ago, about a week after my annual BreastScreen mammogram, I was called and told that there had been some changes in my right breast compared to the previous mammogram.

My first reaction was that "It had to come sometime!" as, at almost 66, I was nearing the age at which my mother had been diagnosed with breast cancer. In fact, my mammograms were annual because of this family history. On the other hand, I had detected no changes myself and thought it quite likely that, after examination, I would be given the "all clear."

More detailed mammograms followed, and I was impressed by the expertise that had detected these little marks, which were barely visible to me. I was then told that a "broad needle" biopsy would be necessary. This "broad needle" biopsy, where one lies facedown on a couch or examination table and lets the breast drop through an aperture for the procedure [see Figure 1.8], sounded nasty, but I was assured that it wouldn't be painful—and so it turned out. The doctor told me that she had left some clips in the breast to indicate where the calcification was.

Following these procedures, I was calmly told that I had DCIS, which was not yet cancer but, left to develop, could become cancer. When I returned to our car, where my husband awaited me, he was shaken to see me coming with a large manila envelope and immediately realized that this wasn't "all clear" as it had been every previous year. However, he set about ringing a friend who had recently had a breast operation to find the best surgeon for me. It seemed to help him that he was able to do something constructive.

I made an appointment with the surgeon, who was able to answer some of my queries: Did the fact that there were multiple occurrences of calcification mean that these were "secondaries" (i.e., had some cancer metastasized)? The answer was no, it was just in the one breast. My other query was: If conditions were right for DCIS in the right breast, wouldn't there be a high probability for it to occur in the left breast also? I was told that, on the contrary, this was rare.

I opted to have just the affected area removed as the DCIS seemed to have been caught at the early stages. Preparation for surgery required the insertion of a wire into my breast to indicate where the occurrences were. This rather horrified me, and in fact looked bad, with a bit of bleeding, but my memory of it was not of a great deal of pain, just discomfort.

The operation was soon over—it was day surgery only—and I was told to remove the dressing the following day. The wound was very neat, and as became apparent in the months to come, it is scarcely noticeable, being around the contour of my nipple.

At my subsequent appointment, the surgeon confirmed that all the DCIS had been removed and referred me to an oncologist, who booked me in for radiotherapy in about six weeks' time. Here again, I had much to learn: I did not lose my hair and, in fact, had no ill effects at all. The radiotherapy was carefully calibrated for my case and each treatment (given daily, Monday to Friday for six weeks) consisted of several bursts of radiation, together lasting less than thirty seconds. I was able to carry on all my normal activities around the radiotherapy and do not remember feeling extra tired.

I continue to have annual mammograms and have had no further recurrence of the DCIS or of cancer. My experience has given me confidence in the medical staff I have dealt with. I am reminded of my mother's comments after her double mastectomy, "I have decided that there are worse things than breast cancer!" With the early diagnosis of DCIS, our prospects are even better.

CONTROL POINT #2

HOW DO I FIND THE RIGHT TREATMENT TEAM?

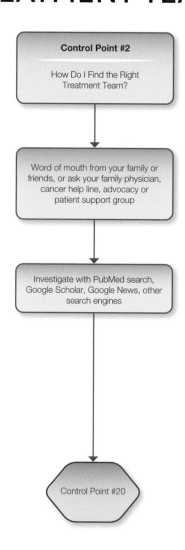

How Do I Find the Right Treatment Team?

It's very scary when you find out you have this "alphabet" diagnosis called DCIS or ductal carcinoma in situ. Your whole life stops; nothing else matters all of a sudden. Your work takes second priority, you often can't hear what is going on around you, and a lot of the information you receive from doctors, nurses, and well-meaning friends and relatives often goes in one ear and out the other. You lose control, and decisions may be made for you in a hurry. Believe me, at this point, there are times when it seems like a mountain has just landed on the road you're traveling, and you simply can't climb over it: lots of doctors; waiting rooms; information; searching the Web and obtaining information from various support groups, help lines, or outdated books in your local library.

I want to hold you by the hand and show you how to walk around this mountain and get to the other side after your diagnosis and treatment of DCIS.

I hope that when you were told about your DCIS, you had somebody with you. It is particularly hard being told on your own. Take somebody with you whenever you're reaching key crossroads, when you need to make a choice, or when you're receiving important results such as your pathology reports after your surgery. Give your support person this book to read, as well, so they also have the knowledge to help you.

Knowledge helps you gain control by understanding nearly as much as your doctor about DCIS in these vital first weeks after your diagnosis. These are the critical steps to take on day one to regain some control over your situation:

- Remember that DCIS is not a "medical emergency"—taking a few extra days to ensure that you get the right information and treatment won't harm you.

- Understand your choices and don't get rushed into a decision you don't feel comfortable with. Find the best option for your own individual situation.

- Find a doctor who can deliver that option safely and efficiently without significant waiting times.

- Take notes, ask your support person to be a note taker, or take a digital recorder with you.

- Ask to get a copy of letters or other correspondence doctors may send to each other.

- Keep a copy of all your test results and correspondence in ascending chronological order in one of those folders with lots of clear plastic sheets.

- Keep a copy of details of your insurance company, policy number, contact telephone numbers, health care cards, and a log of important dates including your consultations, dates of surgery, when you started and finished radiation therapy, and dates when you started or finished any hormonal treatment.

- Write your telephone number on all your X-rays, as they often get lost or left behind in hospitals.

- Inquire about any support groups, taking into account that breast cancer groups may not be right for you and can be scary.

- Consider keeping a journal or blog of your thoughts, experiences, and feelings.

- See if your team includes a breast care nurse, who is usually more accessible than the doctor, and ask for his or her business card or contact number.

- Ask for a business card from all the professionals you meet.

- Better still, find a doctor who works in a team—a **surgeon**, a **radiation oncologist**, and sometimes a **medical oncologist**. The team should work closely with other specialists, such as a plastic surgeon and a geneticist, and have access to expert nurses and other allied health staff.

- If you live outside a large city, it is of course harder to see the whole team before your surgery. Seek an opinion from a surgeon who has networks with a cancer center, or if you can afford the time, money, extra stress, and inconvenience of leaving your home, seek a second opinion.

- Be prepared to take control of your destiny, particularly during follow-up as most doctors don't have the time to provide you the emotional support you need.

Not having information and waiting around for your appointments can be very demoralizing and isolating at times. It gets better.

Understanding the Mumbo Jumbo

Several years ago, I was involved in some psychological research with the National Breast Cancer Centre in Sydney about what women understand after a diagnosis of DCIS. We recruited twenty-six patients from across Sydney who had been diagnosed and treated by sixteen different surgeons. The patients were mostly interviewed within two years of their original diagnosis and treatment (De Morgan et al. 2002).

Five small focus group sessions were held to explore the women's experience of being diagnosed with DCIS. The findings in the following five areas were, in my mind, not unexpected.

1. Response to the diagnosis: Most women were obviously shocked as they had no symptoms and were detected by an abnormal mammogram. Most women have never heard of DCIS before a mammogram compared to invasive breast cancer, which is always in the news.

2. Understanding the diagnosis: Women were often confused about whether or not they had invasive breast cancer that could result in death, hence the title of the publication: "Well, Have I Got Cancer or Haven't I?" Many women thought they had cancer. Others were told by their surgeon that it was "benign." One patient's surgeon said, "Yes, it's definitely cancer. It's in the milk ducts, which is all just contained." Although what the surgeon said above was correct in a biological sense, you can imagine how confused this poor lady would have felt. Indeed, the cells look like cancer cells, but because they haven't invaded through the wall of the duct it is *not* cancer but precancer or precancerous.

3. Satisfaction with information: Most women in the focus group interviews expressed dissatisfaction with the amount of information, both written and verbal, they received about DCIS: "They gave you plenty of stuff on breast cancer and radiotherapy and all those sorts of things; but on the specifics of actual DCIS, there wasn't a lot." One woman was quoted as saying: "But you still feel at the end of the day, it's inconclusive. Well, I feel like I'm on some kind of seesaw of medical incompetence."

4. Satisfaction with the level of involvement in treatment decision making: The study also found that the difficulty in treatment decision making and the confusion about the nature of DCIS was made worse for some women by the use of mastectomy as a treatment option for DCIS. Many women considered this to indicate that their disease was an invasive condition. Some women were further confused by the promotion of breast conserving surgery (lumpectomy) to treat invasive breast cancer when they were advised to have a mastectomy. One participant said, "I am having a mastectomy for this precancerous condition. Am I really overreacting here, or what's going on?"

5. Satisfaction with support services: At the time of the study, there were no support groups for women with DCIS. This is probably still true of most centers today.

Another study was published with a larger sample of 144 women diagnosed with and treated for DCIS within the past twelve months (De Morgan et al. 2011). The authors again found that communication could have been better, particularly in the area of differentiating DCIS from invasive cancer that can spread (only 46% satisfied), risks to the patients' daughter(s) (56% satisfied), and risk of DCIS coming back (34% satisfied).

The authors also studied the degree of worry women had after a diagnosis of DCIS. They found that 75% of women worried about breast cancer coming in the other breast, 66% worried that DCIS or invasive breast cancer could come back in the chest wall region after a mastectomy or in the breast after conservation, and over 40% still worried about dying from breast cancer or cancer coming back in another part of the body.

Doctors' Understanding of DCIS

Apart from the study in Australia, a large survey of 296 health professionals was performed in the U.K. about their understanding of DCIS. The study included ninety surgeons, and twenty-eight oncologists with the remainder being other types of doctors and nurses (Kennedy et al. 2009). Of concern, there was marked discrepancy in how these groups perceived DCIS. About 40% of all non-oncologist health professionals (including surgeons who treat the disease) described DCIS as "cancer" compared to less than 5% of oncologists.

A similar study from Harvard University in the U.S. found that nearly 80% of U.S. physicians in the study found decision making for DCIS as difficult (36%) or more difficult (42%) than for women with invasive breast cancer. Less busy doctors reported that DCIS posed more risk to patients' overall long-term health than busier doctors who saw women with DCIS more frequently. This again reaffirms the importance of seeing doctors with experience in this breast disease, who work in a team and have more confidence in the biology and treatment of DCIS. Of concern, like in the U.K., 63% of physicians reported that they "always" or "almost always" refer to DCIS as cancer and 21% "never" or "almost never" refer to DCIS as cancer (Partridge et al. 2008).

Lydia's Story

Lydia was an attractive, outgoing 52-year-old woman when she went to a public screening mammogram facility and was discovered to have a 60 mm area of microcalcifications in the outer part of her left breast. A core biopsy revealed high-grade DCIS. She was referred to a local surgeon who advised a mastectomy. The staff of the screening unit also strongly advised a mastectomy. She asked her general practitioner for a second opinion from our team after she found us on the Internet and started doing her own research. Her breasts were a C-cup, and we knew there was enough normal breast tissue to try and get around this area of microcalcification.

We arranged for an MRI to help us plan her surgery and inserted two hookwires at either end of the calcification. The MRI, surprisingly, showed the area to be about half the size of the area on the mammogram. The suspect area was removed and showed high-grade DCIS with no invasive cancer and clear margins. The area measured 27 mm (instead of 60 mm as appeared on the mammogram), and some of the surrounding spots of calcium were, in fact, benign. Her margins were clear, meaning that there was some healthy tissue around the area of DCIS. She was now ready to start her radiation. Taking control often means having the courage to seek a second opinion.

This sort of data is depressing as a treating doctor when you know that (1) over 99% of women will not die of breast cancer after treatment for DCIS; (2) the risk of breast cancer appearing in the opposite healthy breast is less than 5 in 100 for most women; and (3) the long-term chance of some sort of a recurrence in the breast is less than 8–10% after a lumpectomy and radiation and less than 2% after a mastectomy.

The challenge for me in the rest of the book is to objectively present the data to make you feel comfortable with your treatment decision and the fact that you are more than likely to survive DCIS.

It Pays to Do Some Research about Your Doctors

Based on the research above from Australia, the U.S., and the U.K., it is vital that you now understand the "aerial view" of your treatment journey by reading the "Control Points" flow charts at the start of each chapter. Refer back to these frequently when you come to important steps or decision points.

This should not turn into a doctor-bashing exercise. Rather, it's about you understanding the medical aspects of the disease, what is possible and what is not possible, and what treatments can and cannot be given safely in a particular situation. Do your research, but don't go overboard. Be particularly guided by your family doctor, who knows you and your medical history.

Do a Google search of the doctor to whom you've been referred. See what articles he or she has written. This will provide a guideline of a doctor's specific interests and expertise and may give you a clue to whether he or she works as part of a team. One quick way of doing this is via **Google Scholar**. Go to www.Google.com and click "more," then find the Google Scholar link in the drop-down menu.

To find some of my articles, type in "John Boyages" with the quotation marks, as this gives a more exact search. Do the same thing in Google and type in your doctor's name in quotation marks. Here is what happens: Google Scholar found 155 articles. It doesn't pick them all up, but it does give you a quick understanding. When I typed in "John Boyages" + DCIS, it retrieved thirty-seven articles in which I spoke specifically about DCIS (Figure 2.1).

Here is another way to do a search on your doctor's publications that is probably more accurate. **PubMed** was developed at the National Library of Medicine (NLM), located at the U.S.

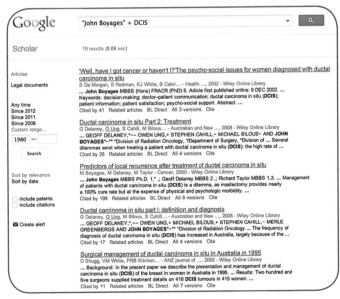

Figure 2.1 A Google Scholar search is a good way to start investigating your doctor.

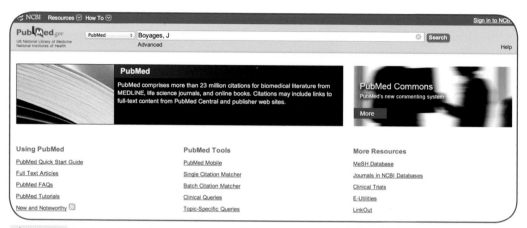

Figure 2.2 A PubMed search on your doctor will show you most of their published work.

National Institutes of Health (NIH). It indexes all of the journals in **MEDLINE** and many other citations. MEDLINE contains citations from 1950 to the present, with a focus on the biomedical sciences. Approximately 5,200 journals published in the United States and more than eighty other countries have been selected and are currently indexed for MEDLINE and are, therefore, included in PubMed. It contains 22 million citations.

To start a PubMed search, type in www.ncbi.nlm.nih.gov/pubmed (Figure 2.2).

Type the author's name into the search bar at the top of the page and click "Search". When I did this search in December 2012, I had 101 publications indexed in PubMed. Remember, this is not all of an individual's publications as some journals are not indexed in MEDLINE or PubMed, particularly those outside the U.S., but it does give you a guideline on what (and when) they have published.

But please remember that this is only a guideline. There are some really fabulous doctors who are just busy being good doctors and attending education updates at conferences who do not have the time or writing skills required to publish. Some doctors who are very prolific in publications may not necessarily be the best technical surgeons or best communicators. Do your research, but keep it in perspective. You need a doctor who can look after you well and keep up with the latest information, and who is prepared to listen to *your* needs.

Finding a Doctor

Most patients are referred from their family physician to a breast surgeon. In some countries, there are directories of doctors. One patient I treated asked her radiologist who he'd refer his wife to for treatment.

Often, your national cancer organization is aware of any available directories. In the U.S., consider going to an NCI (National Cancer Institute)-designated cancer center or a center affiliated with a university medical school. There are also many community cancer programs where doctors are part of a **multidisciplinary team** that includes surgeons, oncologists, radiologists, breast care nurses, and many other team members. If you're not comfortable with your doctor or team, seek a second opinion. The American Cancer Society may be able to help find you a team that will suit your circumstances. They can be contacted at 1-800-ACS-2345. They can also help with support groups. In Australia, the Cancer Council helpline can be contacted at 13-11-20.

Don't forget to encourage at least one designated friend or family member to read this book and attend your appointments with you. It's quite easy to "go blank" during a consultation and not really hear what is being said when you're still in a state of shock. What's really important at this point is family and friends who will support you. At the point of diagnosis, most women I see are shocked and confused about DCIS. But remember, if you have pure DCIS (with no areas of invasive breast cancer), you will have a very, very high cure rate after your treatment.

CONTROL POINT #2 – HOW DO I FIND THE RIGHT TREATMENT TEAM?

WARNING
Understand your choices and don't get rushed into a decision you don't feel comfortable with.

TIP
Take a few extra days to find the right team. Find a doctor who works in a team that includes a surgeon and a radiation oncologist.

REMEMBER
DCIS is not a medical emergency. It pays to do some research about your doctors.

Penny's Story

When I was diagnosed with DCIS, I originally went to my GP who suggested a surgeon, Dr X.

I found him a little intimidating, so I went back to my GP with some names given to me by the screening unit. I found that the surgeon did not have enough time to answer my questions.

It was a little scary going back to my doctor to get another referral as I felt he may have thought I had lost trust in him (my GP). I just said, "The surgeon and I didn't hit it off," and my GP said, "I'll keep that in mind for next time I see a patient with DCIS."

The surgeon I saw eventually worked in a team and had a very supportive breast care nurse who connected me with an oncology team in Sydney.

My advice is to get as much information as you can about your treatment team before your surgery.

CONTROL POINT #3

HOW DO I COPE WITH MY FAMILY AND FRIENDS?

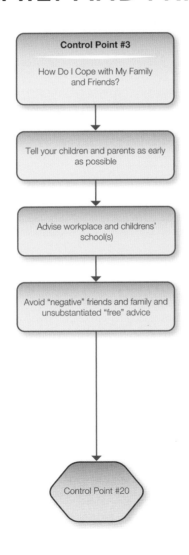

Control Point #3

How Do I Cope with My Family and Friends?

↓

Tell your children and parents as early as possible

↓

Advise workplace and childrens' school(s)

↓

Avoid "negative" friends and family and unsubstantiated "free" advice

↓

Control Point #20

3

Breaking Your News to Others

There is absolutely no doubt that this is a tough call. Who do you tell? What can you say? When do you say something? How do you tell someone else "I have DCIS" when even some health professionals have trouble explaining it? What is certain from my experience is that, despite it being precancer, DCIS can cause a lot of distress and most people will simply assume you have "real" or invasive breast cancer.

There's no right way of doing this. "I've been to the doctor today, and they said I might (or do) have a type of change in my breast that is one step before breast cancer." Or, "The mammogram that I had showed tiny specs of calcium which turned out to be DCIS."

Keep it short and sweet, and most people will give you a hug or say, "I'm really sorry to hear that." Have lots of tissues around at this time. It's better to let the tears out—it's very therapeutic. Talk to your partner, husband, relative, or best friend and let them know what's going on. You don't have to bear the shock of your diagnosis alone. If you have children, talk to them about your disease.

Talk to your family, preferably in person. This is often difficult, and some family members and friends really don't know what to say. Some people, in fact, may stop calling you. They probably think you have a serious type of cancer. This can hurt but don't be too hard on them. It's often just a reaction to their own mortality; or they may not want to upset you or get in your way while you're undergoing treatment.

One particular challenge is talking to other patients at the hospital about your condition. They may have invasive breast cancer requiring chemotherapy and have better access to support services. One of my patients said to me once, "I feel like a fraud. I'm told I don't have breast cancer, but I had to face the same decision about whether or not I needed to lose my breast." Others say, "I'm lucky to have caught it early," and are grateful for that, as detecting the disease early gives many women confidence. Others feel confused about the whole condition and its treatment. Don't place any extra pressure on yourself. Just be positive that you took the right steps to have regular mammograms and have a change like DCIS picked up before it progressed to invasive breast cancer.

Telling Your Children

Ensure open communication. Children usually know something is going on. They can see it in your face. Sit down with them after you've seen the doctor and tell them you need to investigate the abnormality on your mammogram, and things will be all right after you have your treatment. Nobody knows what's around the corner for any of us, so trying to give hope to your children is important to everyone's sense of well-being.

Children are very intuitive, and they know when something is wrong. The problem with not telling them you have a breast problem is that they may instead think that you're having marriage difficulties or that they're a part of the problem, and they won't realize that you're only trying to protect them.

They will certainly pick up on the whispered conversations between adults so, at some point, it's important to sit down with them. It's better to do this as a group so they can all get the same information at the same time. Before talking with your children, talk with your doctor or your breast care nurse and, of course, with your partner to decide what you will and will not say. Perhaps even practice the wording that you'll use. I find that the best approach is to keep things very simple and just see what questions your children ask.

Let them know you have something wrong in your breast, and the area (of DCIS) or the breast needs to removed. Let them know you are going to be all right. Once you know that you are dealing with DCIS, you can say something like, "I have something funny in my breast that needs to be taken out by a surgeon" or, "I will need to go to the hospital every day to have a special treatment to stop "it" coming back." You know your child, and the language you use will vary by their age. At any age, it is best to be upfront about the whole thing no matter how much it hurts you to let them know what is wrong.

Each child behaves differently. Some become very quiet; others become more cuddly and clingy and may want to sleep in bed with you; and others may develop behavioral problems. Give them opportunities to talk about your cancer and your treatment—even with other friends or relatives or schoolmates.

Speak to the school counselor so they'll be more understanding if your child finds it difficult to concentrate at school. Of course, you have to maintain normal discipline and try to keep the family together as much as possible during what may be a very difficult treatment program but always keep them informed.

It's important to continue your child's routine and still drive them to and from school, take them to activities, and spend time with them. Keeping up the routine as much as practically possible is very comforting and reassuring to them. It can be hard when you feel tired from your treatments. Perhaps spend time with them doing less strenuous activities such as watching television, reading a book,

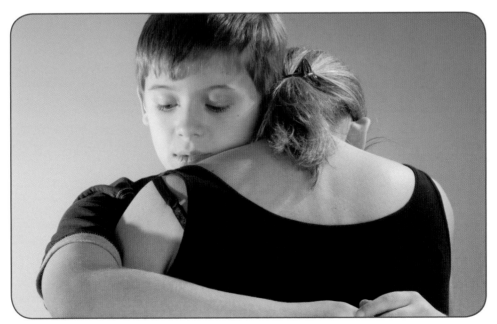

Talking to your children is hard but essential.

or watching one of their favorite movies. Sometimes, depending on the type of surgery you've had, showing them your scar may be important in the healing process.

Some children come along to radiation therapy treatments, particularly when they are on school vacation and you are having a five- or six-week course of radiation therapy. Most staff members are happy to watch the kids while you're having your treatment, and this tends to demystify the whole situation for the children.

With very young children, it's important that they realize that your DCIS is not their fault. It didn't occur because they accidentally bumped your breast or caused you stress from their behavior. In summary, a parent's dilemma is the balance between protecting the child versus enabling understanding. Children need information to be truthful yet hopeful, and they need reassurance about ongoing love and stability, whatever the outcome.

Talking with and Managing Teenagers

Teenagers are probably the hardest group to deal with, particularly the boys. They can go quiet and just ignore the whole situation. You may find this quite disturbing, but just try to give them time, some hugs, and tell them you're going to be all right.

Make sure you still have time to go to their sports or activities and keep up their routine. Teenage boys may find the whole thing embarrassing. They may feel torn between being supportive and wanting to hang with their friends and stay cool and rebellious. Although this can be difficult, it's best to keep the conversation light or get the boy's father or a close friend or mentor to talk to him about your diagnosis.

Teenage girls may become anxious because they feel they will automatically get DCIS or breast cancer too. It's important to reassure them that most breast cancers do not occur in people who have a family history of the disease.

Don't be too hard on your teenagers. Give them some space and keep answering their questions. But remember, it's not enough to talk to them once and then not talk to them again about the situation. Tell them when there has been a change in your treatment plan, when things go right, or if things don't go as well as expected.

It is also important not to put too much pressure on teenagers, for example, by expecting them to clean up their room when they've never cleaned their room before. Kids want you "back to normal" as quickly as possible, and I find that it's important for you as well to be "back to normal" as quickly as possible after your diagnosis. This includes going to work.

Dealing with Your Partner

Like women, many male (or female) partners will be shocked by a diagnosis of DCIS. Men commonly have difficulty concentrating; they can't sleep and experience feelings of loss and sadness. Traditionally, men are the "protectors," and suddenly they're facing a challenge in which they often feel helpless and sometimes very isolated. It is a problem they can't just go out and "fix."

Although DCIS is not life threatening, there is a lot of fear—particularly at first when you are not sure what is going on. You still may not have the results of your biopsy, or you may be concerned that some invasive cancer may be detected once all the DCIS is removed surgically.

Petra's Story

After I was told at the hospital I had DCIS, I went straight home with my husband and let my four- and seven-year-old children know that I had "ABCD" disease which was a type of precancer in my breast. I told them that because grandma had breast cancer, I started to have my breast checks from the age of 40, and a change was found in my breast before it became cancer.

I am so thankful that the mammogram picked it up so early, and I told my children that, apart from daily radiation treatment for six weeks, life would be going on as normal.

My four-year-old daughter loved coming into the radiation department where the staff always made a fuss of her. She cried when I finished my treatment.

That was ten years ago, and my son will be sitting for his final high school exams this year.

The research that I presented above, no doubt, shows that despite your doctor's good intentions (telling you all about precancer or DCIS), patients are still very fearful about their future. Yet many men feel they cannot mention this fear because saying so might be "negative."

Many men are challenged by parental, employment, domestic, and financial changes that come about when a woman is diagnosed with DCIS. The distress and practical support needs of caretakers are frequently overlooked and need to be acknowledged, particularly because caretakers have to deal with their own response and distress as well as yours. Men may also find it difficult to talk to you about sex especially since it's the last thing you may feel like at the moment.

Some men provide outstanding support while others get "too involved" and overprotective, which can be frustrating. I have also seen men just walk out on their partners. So, it's critical to keep communicating with each other during this difficult time. I've also heard of many men falling in love and having deep and meaningful relationships with women who have beaten breast cancer or DCIS. Getting DCIS of the breast does not mean no future relationships! This equally applies to female partners.

It's best to read this section together with your partner and try at all times to talk about your mutual feelings. This is often not a natural thing for males to do, so women, who are generally more experienced sharing their feelings, should try to be patient with them.

Men may be embarrassed to talk about your diagnosis at work. In some cultures, it may bring "shame" to the family. In others, the woman is expected to keep doing everything "as normal" as possible around the house, at work, and in the bedroom!

It can be very, very hard, but most women show enormous strength and get through this difficult post-diagnosis phase. Men also fear asking for attention at a time when they believe their partner or loved one should be the focus of attention. Men who fail to speak out or seek emotional support may experience higher levels of distress.

But remember, everyone gets through this phase. Treatment always finishes, appointments stop, and it's very important that life goes on, including intimacy and short escapes. Plan little breaks away—weekend vacations (even one night away) without the children—and keep on talking with each other.

Dealing with Friends

All of us have different levels of friendships. We may have a very close friend with whom we can express our true thoughts and feelings. Have a "cuppa" with your best friend and tell him or her what's going on.

If friends stop calling you, either ignore them or give them a call and say, "You've probably heard that I've been diagnosed with an abnormality in my breast. It's called DCIS, which is precancer. I'm going to be all right, and I'd be very grateful if you could pop in and see me or run an errand or prepare a meal." This may break the ice, or you may decide to leave friends alone for the moment if they don't call you.

Another option is just to be upfront about the diagnosis and leave it there, and see who emerges to offer a helping hand. Some patients I know just announce it to their friends on Facebook. Often, there'll be new friends made at this time. It's another important chapter of your life and, just as you made new friends when your children started school or you started a new job, you will find new friends who understand your journey with breast cancer—often because they are going through it too.

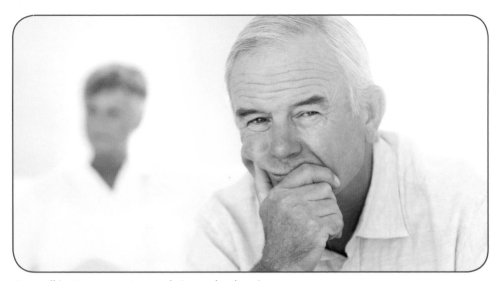

Keep talking to your partner and give each other time.

Some of my patients have friends that always seem to upset them or say the wrong thing. They may be giving "free advice" and talking to you about the latest herb, potion, or lotion that may help with your condition. They may think you have breast cancer and can't really understand the difference between DCIS and breast cancer. Listen to them, but don't become too engaged with this behavior.

I particularly worry about the "friends" who tell you of other patients who died of breast cancer. They link the death to a particular treatment the patient may or may not have had (such as breast conservation or a mastectomy), when in fact it had no connection to their treatment at all from a medical or scientific perspective. Thank your friends for their advice. Maybe say, "I feel a bit overwhelmed by all the advice I'm getting at the moment, but thank you anyway. For now, I'm going to follow my doctor's advice."

Dealing with Your Employer

The reality is that many of my patients continue to work while having radiation therapy for DCIS. If you have a mastectomy, you will also need four to six weeks to recover both physically and emotionally. Your emotions will be quite raw at first.

At the outset, you really don't know how you will feel or react. Don't give up your job just because you have DCIS. The decision to stop working will depend on lots of factors, including where you live, where you work, where your treatment is to be undertaken, and the complexity of your treatment. Usually, you will be off work for about four to six weeks after your surgery, but you can get back to work after you start radiation once you know how you'll cope with any side effects.

I find that people who stay at work often cope much better than they would sitting at home and just staring at the four walls. Most of my patients find they can usually work during radiation therapy by having their treatment first thing in the morning or by taking the last appointment in the afternoon. You may need to get to bed a little earlier because radiation therapy can cause some fatigue, but not enough to interrupt your normal routine or stop you from working. But if you'd prefer to take sick leave and can afford to stop work for a little while, you now have the perfect excuse to do so.

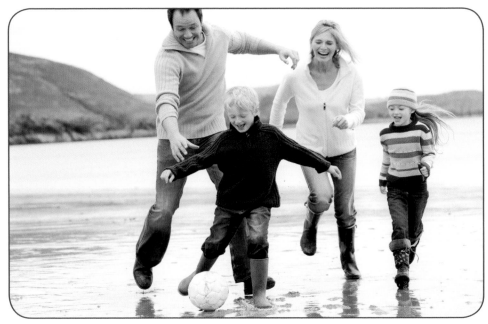

Life usually gets better once your treatment ends. Plan a vacation.

This is why you need to take control and know what's best for you, because you may get conflicting advice. Sometimes, it's from trainees who don't have much experience; sometimes, it's from doctors or other health professionals; and, of course, the Internet can be a challenge with the vast range of information and alternative treatments and solutions you can find there. Take care with the Internet, and look at some of the sites I recommend at the back of this book.

Facing treatment to your breast for DCIS is often the perfect excuse to change aspects of your life or work you don't particularly like for the better. Consider working part-time before resigning, or try to take some paid or unpaid leave. If you really hate your job, maybe this is the time to move on! Plan a vacation after your treatment.

CONTROL POINT #3 – HOW DO I COPE WITH MY FAMILY AND FRIENDS?

WARNING

Avoiding telling your close family, especially your children, about your diagnosis will only add to your stress. Tell them sooner rather than later.

TIP

DCIS is often the perfect excuse to change aspects of your life or work you don't particularly like for the better.

REMEMBER

While there are certainly some storm clouds around, most clouds have a silver lining; and some good nearly always comes out of this illness.

Glenda's Story

Glenda worked in an office in the city. She was having daily radiation treatment close to home, and traveling between the two took about an hour each day. Her treatment was going well and after two weeks of radiation, there were no side effects.

I encouraged her to work throughout her treatment. Ultimately, she decided to take some time off as she found the stress of going to work, cutting into her lunch hour to have treatment, and running off to pick up her children just too hard.

Glenda valued the time on her own to collect her thoughts, get used to her "new normal" self, and have some extra time to spend with the children. Staying at home is not for everyone but don't hesitate to press the "pause" button if the added burden of treatment for DCIS is just too much for now.

PART 2

"GAINING CONTROL"

TAKING CONTROL BEFORE
YOUR SURGERY

WHAT WILL I DO ABOUT MY BREAST?

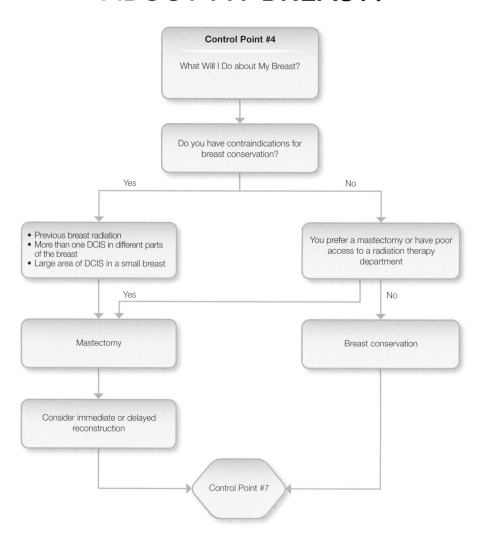

Control Point #4

What Will I Do about My Breast?

Do you have contraindications for breast conservation?

Yes   No

- Previous breast radiation
- More than one DCIS in different parts of the breast
- Large area of DCIS in a small breast

You prefer a mastectomy or have poor access to a radiation therapy department

Yes   No

Mastectomy

Breast conservation

Consider immediate or delayed reconstruction

Control Point #7

A Garden Analogy

Two decisions need to be made, and the first and most important decision is how your breast should be treated. The second, and usually less important, decision is what to do about the lymph glands under your armpit.

Earlier, I mentioned that the breast can be compared to a rosebush in your garden, and the cancer to a weed growing under it (Figure 4.1). The first and more "radical" option is to have the entire breast removed together with the cancer in it—better known as a mastectomy. This is like a gardener removing the whole rosebush, getting out his or her large spade and leaving behind no evidence of the plant or the weed underneath.

The less radical procedure is to remove the cancer with a healthy margin of normal breast tissue—better known as breast conservation. This is like the gardener using a smaller spade and removing just the weed plus a small area of surrounding soil. The problem is that the weed can still come back even though the remaining soil looks clear. To reduce that risk, we need to smother any remaining seeds that may have been left behind when the weed was taken out.

In a garden, we may use a weed mat, or some newspaper or straw mulch, but with DCIS, we use a course of radiation therapy. Without radiation therapy, the risk of the DCIS coming back (either as DCIS or a real cancer, called an invasive cancer) can be as high as 30% over the next five to ten years following a lumpectomy; the risk is 5–10% if radiation is given.

Please, please, please—do not rush this decision! Once the breast is gone, it cannot be put back!

There are two questions that you must answer at this point:

1. Do I have the whole breast removed (this is like removing the whole rosebush)? Or . . .

2. Do I have the abnormal area removed with a lumpectomy (this is like removing the weed along with a small amount of surrounding soil and keeping the rosebush), and then consider having a course of radiation therapy lasting five to six weeks?

You may feel more comfortable with a mastectomy (Figure 4.5), but your surgeon may try to convince you to have a lumpectomy (Figure 4.6). Or your surgeon may be recommending a lumpectomy but your family is pushing you to have a mastectomy. Get all the information then go with your own gut feeling.

Before I go too much further, I'd like to point out the six different parts of the breast that doctors refer to. These parts are the four "quadrants," the "central" part behind the nipple and areola (pigmented

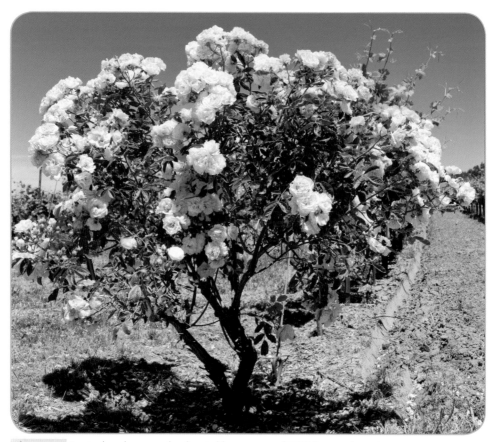

Figure 4.1 A weed under a rosebush—is like an area of DCIS in your breast.

area around your nipple), and the "axillary tail," which is the part of the breast that extends toward your armpit (Figure 4.2). Knowing which quadrant or quadrants your cancer is in is important, particularly if your cancer involves more than one quadrant; a mastectomy may be indicated; or the cancer is behind the nipple (central area), in which case the nipple may need to be removed if you want to keep your breast.

If you found a lump, which is uncommon for DCIS, the surgeon will feel the lump while you're under anesthetic and remove it with a rim of healthy tissue. If your cancer was only found on mammogram or—less frequently—ultrasound and the surgeon cannot feel a lump (which is the more usual situation), then the procedure I mentioned earlier called "wire localization" will be performed by a radiologist usually on the morning of your surgery (Figure 1.13, page 25).

Before I go into the potential situations where it is better for your DCIS to be treated by a mastectomy, I'd like to review the data with you on key research where pathologists and radiologists meticulously worked out the distribution and number of areas of DCIS in women who had undergone a mastectomy. An exceptional study from the Netherlands showed that high-grade DCIS tended to grow in a continuous way without gaps between separate areas (90% of cases), a bit like a patch of grass growing into the soil under the rosebush (Holland 1990).

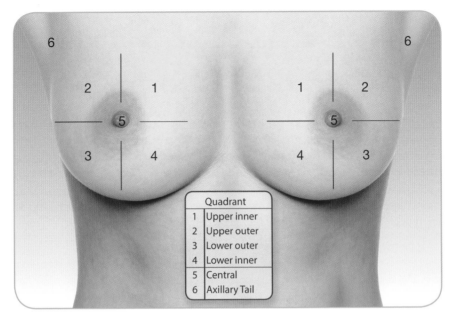

Quadrant	
1	Upper inner
2	Upper outer
3	Lower outer
4	Lower inner
5	Central
6	Axillary Tail

Figure 4.2 Different locations on the breast, called "quadrants".

For low- or intermediate-grade DCIS, it was continuous only in 30% to 45% of cases. However, in most cases, even though there were gaps between the different patches of DCIS, they were found to be small (< 5 mm). This is a bit like having a weed, then some soil, then another weed then the soil in a checkerboard type of pattern. What this means is that for most patients with DCIS, the abnormal area appears to be confined to a segment. This is not to say that the segment may not be large (like the large yellow duct seen in the lower part of Figure D on page 11). So the good news is that if the surgeon can get around the abnormal area with clear margins, you may have a good chance of keeping your breast.

Indications for a Mastectomy

The absolute reasons to have a mastectomy for DCIS are:

- When there is more than one proven area of DCIS in different quadrants of the breast. If there is an area of DCIS, for example, at the eleven o'clock position, 4.0 cm from the right nipple (upper outer quadrant) and another at the five o'clock position, 5.0 cm from the right nipple (lower inner quadrant), then you are probably better off having a mastectomy. This situation is called multicentric DCIS (Figure 4.3). On the other hand, if you have two or more areas of DCIS in the same quadrant that are quite close together as in Figure 4.4 (upper inner quadrant), then there is absolutely no need to have a mastectomy, provided the surgeon can get around both areas with a clear margin. This situation is called **multifocal DCIS.**

- If, as a child or a teenager, you had cancer that required radiation therapy. Some patients with a type of cancer of the lymph glands known as Hodgkin's lymphoma will have had radiation therapy in the past to the breast area that may make subsequent radiation therapy to the breast quite difficult.

- If you just feel more comfortable having a mastectomy than going through five or six weeks of radiation

- If clear margins cannot be obtained after one to three breast conserving procedures. The number of procedures usually depends on the size of your breast.

The relative reasons to have a mastectomy for DCIS are:

- If you have a very large area of DCIS, particularly in a smaller breast. One patient I saw over fifteen years ago had the largest area of DCIS I have ever treated. It spanned an area of about 80 mm (see Ruth's story). I suggested that the surgeon use two hookwires on either side of it (this is called "bracketing"), and he managed to remove it with clear margins. She had very large breasts, which meant that removing the abnormal area did not leave a major cosmetic deformity. I treated her with radiation and she has remained free of disease ever since. Just because an area of DCIS is large, it doesn't necessarily mean you need a mastectomy.

- If you are pregnant, you cannot receive radiation until you have delivered your baby, so a mastectomy may be more appropriate for you. However, given that DCIS is not yet cancer, you can go ahead and have your surgery before your delivery and then have your radiotherapy after the delivery.

- Some preexisting diseases (such as severe scleroderma or rheumatic diseases requiring high-dose steroids) may make you more prone to radiation complications, and a mastectomy may be less complicated.

Having a strong family history of breast cancer is not necessarily an indication for a mastectomy if you have DCIS. Most studies have found that if you have a **first-degree** family history, you may have

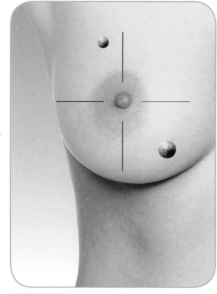

Figure 4.3 Two areas of DCIS in different parts of the breast (multicentric).

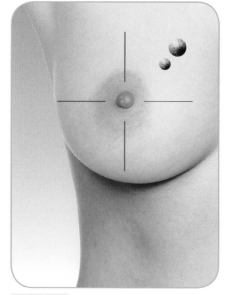

Figure 4.4 Two areas of DCIS close to each other (multifocal).

a slightly higher risk of a recurrence in the breast after a lumpectomy alone or lumpectomy with radiation. A first-degree relative is usually your mother, sister or daughter but rarely may include the males in your family. However, when adjusted for all the other competing factors, family history on its own is less important. One large study from five centers in France of 719 patients showed that— apart from not having radiation—the most significant risk factor was being under the age of 40 at the time of your diagnosis and having the DCIS excised with incomplete margins rather than a family history (Cutuli et al. 2009).

A study from the University of Pennsylvania found that women with DCIS and a first-degree family history had a recurrence rate in the breast, after a lumpectomy and radiation, of 8% at ten years, lower than the 16% for women with no family history (Harris et al. 2000). This study did not find that women under the age of 50 had a higher recurrence rate even with a strong family history. Of note, however, was that the risk of breast cancer on the healthy side was 18% at ten years for those with a strong family history and 8% for those without a family history. The five-year survival rate was not affected by the presence of a family history—it was 100% for those with a family history of breast cancer and 99% for those without a family history.

Some doctors do occasionally recommend removing both breasts in this setting, but there is no evidence that this increases your chance of surviving a future breast cancer although it makes intuitive sense that it could. For invasive breast cancer, most studies have found little or no difference in the chance of cancer coming back after breast conservation for patients with or without the breast cancer gene (Recht 2009).

Nevertheless, I personally find very young patients and those with a very strong family history one of the more difficult groups with DCIS to advise. You may have seen your mother or sister or grand-mother develop breast cancer at a very young age. If they were diagnosed under the age of 50, or if both their breasts were involved, or there is a family history of ovarian cancer, this increases the likelihood of having a breast cancer gene. In this setting, I find it useful to see the genetics team and to have genetic testing. Removing the breast may indeed be the best option for you as it largely prevents future cancer appearing. In the setting where you have the breast cancer gene and now have a curable DCIS, it is worthwhile to seriously consider removing both breasts with a reconstruction using a "skin-sparing" approach that I will describe later. If you are in this situation, make sure you see a team who specializes in women with a strong family history. Our patients are usually seen a few times by both the surgeon and oncologist, who refer them to our psychologist to carefully make the decision one way or the other.

In an excellent collaborative study from the European Union, 236 women with a strong family history and with DCIS or invasive breast cancer on one side underwent a preventative mastectomy on the healthy side and treatment by a mastectomy on the affected side (Evans et al. 2009). Most women had a skin-sparing mastectomy with some sort of reconstruction. About 30% of women also had preserva-tion of their nipple region. The average follow-up was about seven years. About 3% were discovered to have DCIS or invasive breast cancer in the unaffected breast following their prophylactic surgery.

So, it's a tough call as none of us can look into the future. I find that most women in our practice don't rush in and have both breasts taken off if there is only a mild to moderate family history, but we certainly consider it if everyone around them has had breast cancer. If you have DCIS, you have many years of life ahead of you as your disease is very curable. For many women having both breasts removed gives them a sense of relief as their waiting for the time bomb to go off is finally over. For many women with a family history or who are aged under 50 years of age, **tamoxifen** is another option I use to reduce the chance of DCIS or invasive cancer coming back (see "Control Point #17– Do I Need Hormonal Treatment?"). My final words on this are: just proceed slowly and with caution.

The Difference between a Breast Surgeon and a General Surgeon

Surgeons are always trained first as general surgeons, and then they usually specialize in a field such as brain, heart, or breast surgery, particularly if they work in a large hospital or academic university hospital. If you can, consult a breast surgeon who sees and treats breast cancer every single day. Take care if your surgeon spends a lot of his or her week doing gallbladders, hemorrhoids, varicose veins, or colorectal cancer and only operates on the occasional patient with breast cancer. I do, however, exclude very experienced rural surgeons. It's impossible for every country town or small state to have a breast surgeon. My experience of these country surgeons is that they provide exceptional service and work very hard to keep up to date and linked in with experienced breast surgeons by telephone, e-mail, or video conference.

Remember that an experienced general mechanic in the country may still be better than the young Ford mechanic in the city. You can ask the surgeon, "What proportion of your work is breast disease?" Remember that very busy breast surgeons may focus 80–90% of their practice on breast disease and 10% on hormone conditions such as thyroid disease. Some surgeons sub-specialize in cancer operations ("surgical oncologists"), and some may focus on both breast cancer and melanoma (a type of skin cancer). Breast surgeons know about **sentinel node mapping** and the **sentinel node biopsy** technique, explained in the next chapter, and generally work in a team with oncologists.

Remember, a doctor's personality isn't everything (although it helps a lot). Also important is their ability to do nice wounds with stitches under the skin, if possible. These are called **sub-cuticular stitches** (Figure 4.5–4.6) and are preferable to "railroad tracks," or cross-hatching, where the stitches are applied outside the skin at right angles to the main incision. Sub-cuticular stitches dissolve on their own and leave a less obvious scar than external stitches or staples, which need to be removed by your surgeon. Also, your surgeon should be linked in with a cancer treatment team that includes at least a radiation and a medical oncologist.

What Is Oncoplastic Surgery?

Some surgeons are now trained in advanced plastic surgery techniques to reshape the remaining breast after your cancer is removed. This is sometimes referred to as **oncoplastic surgery**. The breast surgeon uses plastic surgical techniques in order to reshape the remaining healthy breast or reconstruct the affected breast after removal of DCIS or breast cancer. It also includes the correction of any imbalance relative to your healthy breast.

Oncoplastic surgery is ideal for women with DCIS who not only have to deal with the diagnosis but also the effect of possible disfiguring surgery to their breast. Surgery still remains the mainstay of treatment for the DCIS.

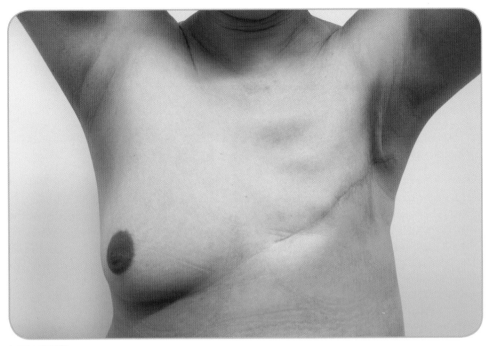

Figure 4.5 A mastectomy scar with dissolving "sub-cuticular" stitches under the skin.

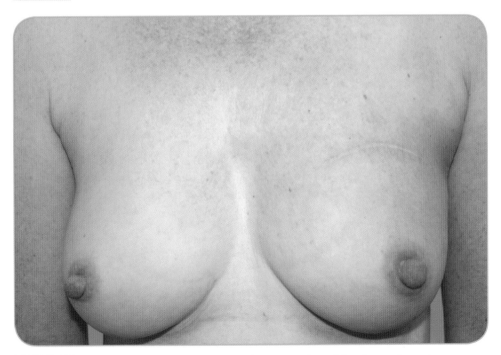

Figure 4.6 A good breast conservation scar with preservation of the shape, shown here four weeks after completing radiation and six months after surgery.

Oncoplastic surgery in the DCIS-affected breast may include the following:

Breast Conservation

- Removing the area of DCIS with a clear margin.

- Using small scars with dissolving stitches under the skin.

- Displacing nearby breast tissue into the defect which is left when your DCIS and surrounding healthy tissue is removed.

- Using breast reduction techniques in order to refashion the whole breast after the DCIS is excised with reduction of the other side to achieve symmetry (Figure 4.7–4.8). Your surgeon may place a non-magnetic clip made from titanium where your cancer started so we know where to give a higher dose of radiation. I have seen a few patients with reduced nipple sensation on both sides after bilateral breast reducing surgery and removal of her cancer on the affected side. Make sure you check with your surgeon about their own experience with this type of surgery.

- Replacing tissue into the surgical defect by moving muscle and skin tissue from elsewhere, for example the **latissimus dorsi muscle (LD) flap** (see "Control Point #7 – If I Have a Mastectomy, What Are My Options for Breast Reconstruction?").

Mastectomy

- Removing all of your breast which leaves behind the skin and some underlying fat and an immediate sub-pectoral **tissue expander** can be placed at the time of surgery and later exchanged for a permanent **implant**. Or, a tissue flap can be used to reconstruct a breast mound (see "Control Point #7 – If I Have a Mastectomy, What Are My Options for Breast Reconstruction?"). In this option the skin and nipple areola is removed from the central part of your breast (with the underlying breast tissue).

- Having a **skin-sparing mastectomy** (SSM) where the breast tissue and the nipple and areola are excised through a small scar thus removing less of the overlying skin. The breast mound is then recreated and the natural shape and contour of the breast is preserved, using a tissue expander followed later by a permanent implant or an immediate permanent implant or tissue flap (Figure 4.9) (Patani & Mokbel 2008).

- As for a skin-sparing mastectomy but with preservation of the nipple and areola (**nipple-sparing mastectomy**) without removal of skin (Figure 4.10).

- Your surgeon may also discuss adjusting the appearance of your other breast to more closely match your treated breast. This is often known as **contralateral symmetrization**. It involves achieving symmetry of the healthy side with a reduction known as a **reduction mammo-plasty** or a breast lift or "mastopexy." **Lipofilling** may be done after breast reconstruction to fix small areas of asymmetry or defects in the shape of the reconstructed breast compared to the normal breast. It can also be done after breast conservation. Fat tissue is removed from

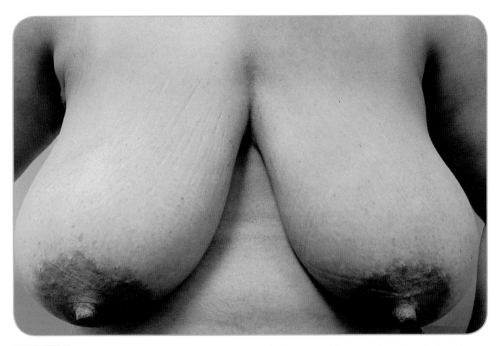

Figure 4.7 A patient with large breasts can have imbalance problems and neck and shoulder pain after a one-sided mastectomy.

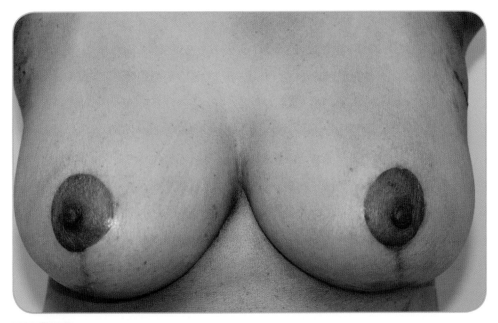

Figure 4.8 A type of oncoplastic surgery where a woman with large breasts (shown in Figure 4.7) had an abnormal area removed from her left breast, followed by a breast reduction of both sides and a left sentinel node biopsy.

another part of the body such as the tummy area, and then injected into the reconstructed breast to improve its shape or fullness. Some doctors were worried that women who had lipofilling would have a higher risk of breast cancer coming back but this has not been found to be the case (Petit et al. 2012).

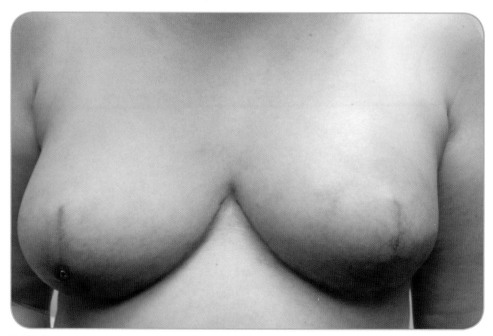

Figure 4.9 A skin-sparing mastectomy on both sides. Preservation of most of the patient's skin of her breast allowed easy placement of a silicon implants at the same time. There was a small amount of delayed wound healing on the right which subsequently healed completely.

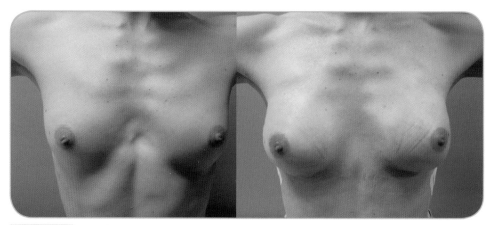

Figure 4.10 A nipple-sparing mastectomy on the right. Preservation of most of the patient's skin of her breast allowed easy placement of a silicone implant at the same time.

Skin-Sparing Mastectomy

The skin-sparing mastectomy (SSM) was first described over 20 years ago in an effort to maximize preservation of the skin of the breast after a mastectomy, to improve the cosmetic appearance of the breast, and to make breast reconstruction easier by having more tissue to work with (Toth & Lappert 1991). It typically involves removal of the entire breast and nipple-areola complex while preserving the skin envelope and the natural curvature under your breast (the **inframammary fold**).

Because less skin is removed, research has looked at the chance of finding residual breast tissue or even disease under the skin that is left behind after a skin-sparing mastectomy. In one study, the chance of finding residual breast tissue was almost 60% and finding residual disease was 10% (Torresan et al. 2005). Despite this, with well-selected patients the chance of a recurrence after a skin-sparing mastectomy is very low. Tokin et al. (2012) reported on five studies involving 368 patients, of whom four patients had recurrence (1.1%). Most of these studies had short observation periods of less than five years. This rate is likely to go up a little with time. For example, we found a recurrence rate of 3.3% for 299 patients with DCIS treated by a conventional mastectomy with follow-up times of at least ten years (Stuart et al. 2011). In a very large study of skin-sparing mastectomy from the Emory University Hospital of 223 patients with DCIS treated by skin-sparing mastectomy and an average follow-up of seven years, recurrences developed in eleven patients (5.1%), including the breast region (3.3%), adjacent lymph nodes (0.9%), or in other parts of the body (0.9%) (Carlson et al. 2007).

Usually after a skin-sparing mastectomy, because of the amount of skin left behind, the so-called "skin-envelope," reconstruction needs to take place either with an expander followed by a silicone implant at a later date or an immediate silicone implant as in Figure 4.9. Or, for some patients with larger breasts, a flap with some normal skin and muscle tissue can be used (see "Control Point # 7 – What Are My Options for Breast Reconstruction?"). A variant of a skin-sparing mastectomy is a "skin-reducing mastectomy" used for larger breasted women, which is like a combination of a breast reduction and a reconstruction with an immediate implant.

Radiation therapy may still be indicated after these types of procedures and this may cause some thickening around your implant and some asymmetry. The indications for post-mastectomy radiation are discussed in "Control Point #16 – Do I Need Radiation Therapy?"

Complications after a skin-sparing mastectomy include infection, other wound problems or loss of the implant. There is a higher risk of delayed wound healing with skin-reducing mastectomy than with other mastectomy types because the blood supply needs to be distributed to a larger portion of skin (see right breast in Figure 4.9). For the standard skin- or nipple-sparing mastectomy, wound healing is usually not a problem, because, in fact, the incisions used are smaller than that of a standard mastectomy. Implant loss has been reported to be on average around 14% (Kobraei et al. 2012).

Nipple-Sparing Mastectomy

Nipple-sparing mastectomy is a variety of skin-sparing mastectomy where the entire skin of the breast is preserved, including the nipple-areola complex (Figure 4.10). The ducts inside of the nipple (its "core") are usually removed. Nipple-sparing mastectomy is particularly suitable for women with smaller breasts and often the other breast is enlarged with an implant at the same time. Often both sides are done at the same time, particularly for women with a very strong family history (Figure 4.10). This is still possible with larger-breasted women, but nipple-sparing mastectomy has been considered safe for women with small, solitary tumors located away from the nipple or when a mastectomy is done as a preventative measure. For instance, some women may have a skin-sparing mastectomy on their breast affected by DCIS and, because of an increased risk on the other side due, for example, to a strong family history, may have a nipple-sparing mastectomy on the healthy side to reduce their future risk of cancer developing. Alternatively, some women with a very strong family history of breast cancer and diagnosed DCIS may choose to have bilateral skin-sparing mastectomies with nipple removal on both sides (Figure 4.9).

As mentioned earlier, DCIS naturally follows the breast ducts that stop or emerge at the nipple. In "Control Point #8", I will also discuss Paget's disease of the nipple, which is a situation where the DCIS involves the main ducts and even the outside of the nipple and the areola. A concern, therefore, is the possibility of leaving DCIS behind if the nipple is preserved.

A review paper about nipple-sparing mastectomy examined all the publications, which studied nipple involvement for women who had undergone a mastectomy (Rusby et al. 2010). The authors found that 13 studies contained a minimum of 100 patients per study and over 4,500 patients total. The average incidence of nipple involvement was 14% (range, 6–31%). These studies are not all alike and vary not only by the type of patients who were included (ranging from those with early to more advanced disease) but also the pathology technique used to examine the nipple.

Rusby et al. (2008), with investigators from the Massachusetts General Hospital, has developed a method of estimating the risk of nipple involvement. Her studies were based on 130 women who'd had a mastectomy for invasive cancer or DCIS. Of note, 75% of the patients either had pure DCIS or had DCIS as part of an invasive cancer.

Use this Web link to estimate your risk of nipple involvement:
www.lifemath.net/cancer/breastcancer/nipplecalc/index.php

It's hard to give an exact cut-off of distance from the nipple but the above calculator suggests that if you have an area of microcalcification (proven by a core biopsy to be DCIS) that measures under 2 cm and is at least 3 cm from the nipple, then the chance of nipple involvement is around 20%. I know that many surgeons are doing this procedure for tumors as close as 1 cm to the nipple.

One large group from the US initially recommended a nipple-sparing mastectomy only after a pre-operative breast MRI showed no abnormality within 2 cm of the nipple (Wijayanayagam et al. 2008). However, as their experience evolved, they now only use an MRI in cases where the tumor is close to the nipple on clinical examination or mammography; if preoperative MRI demonstrates no clear tumor involvement of the nipple or areola, patients are still eligible for this technique, even if the tumor lies within 1 cm of the nipple region (Peled 2012). In contrast to the calculator, this study, led by Laura Esserman, found that the tissue and ducts behind the nipple had disease present in only 3 out of every 100 patients (3%).

Another drawback of this technique is the chance of the nipple losing its blood supply and dying off ("necrosis"). It is likely that the risk is higher if you continue to smoke, if you are older, or if you have vascular disease—all of which can affect the blood supply and healing. Some researchers have found that nipple necrosis was more common when an incision was made centrally around the areola (**periareolar incision**) compared to a scar in the outer half of the breast (Regolo et al. 2008). Others have found that using an expander (which slowly stretches the skin and nipple) rather than a permanent fixed volume implant improved nipple survival (Wijayanayagam et al. 2008).

In the review article, Tokin et al. (2012) reported on 14 studies which treated patients with a nipple-sparing mastectomy. Out of 2,406 patients 257 (10.7%) developed some or total loss of the nipple. In total, 66 patients (2.7%) lost their entire nipple due to it dying off from a lack of blood supply. Ask your surgeon about what his or her rates of nipple necrosis are and how many he or she has done.

In Laura Esserman's study, once their technique was refined, nipple necrosis occurred in 2 out of every 100 patients (one complete and one partial) (1.8%), and necrosis of the overlying mastectomy skin occurred in 11 patients out of every 100 (11.3%). Complications requiring removal of the implant occurred in 8 out of every 100 women (8.4%) (Peled 2012).

Normal nipple sensitivity is very unusual after these procedures. Some sensation in the surrounding skin may be possible in many women and only a few nipples remain potentially erectile. The cosmetic results from a nipple-sparing mastectomy can be excellent (Figure 4.10) but you may appear unbalanced if some sort of lift is not done on the other side.

Radiation to the skin of your new breast may be required and this can tighten your skin a little (and sometimes a lot) causing more asymmetry and increases the risk of implant loss.

I have seen a few patients with disastrous cosmetic results from surgeons who really didn't have the expertise to do this type of procedure. If you are considering this type of surgery, make sure you see a surgeon who has a lot of experience in this technique and, more importantly, works in a multidisciplinary team. If your case is complicated, for whatever reason, it's often worthwhile seeing other team members such as a plastic surgeon, breast care nurse, radiation oncologist, and psychologist before your surgery. Remember, it's not an emergency and DCIS is still not cancer so you have time to reach the right decision for you.

A very good study from Italy restricted nipple-sparing mastectomy for patients whose tumors were located at least 1 cm beyond the edge of the areola. All patients received radiation to the nipple and areola region at the time of the operation. The study looked at the psychological consequences affecting patients whose nipple was preserved in a nipple-sparing mastectomy versus patients who lost their nipple and had it artificially reconstructed later. The investigators found that patients treated with nipple-sparing mastectomy had a more positive perception of themselves, particularly when being seen naked. Their study also showed that patients who preserved their nipple felt less mutilated regarding their breast (Didier et al. 2009).

So, it's not that straightforward, and expertise for these types of operations vary. What is needed is a very careful discussion with a breast and/or a reconstructive surgeon to determine your potential to have one of these more advanced potentially one-stage procedures. Broadly speaking, the surgeons I work with consider the ideal patient to be one who does not have any oncological contraindication to a nipple-sparing mastectomy such as advanced cancer with skin involvement or disease very close to the nipple. This ideal patient would be a non-smoker, non-diabetic, unlikely to require post-mastectomy radiation with no underlying chronic disorders (such as diabetes or rheumatoid arthritis), be no greater than a C-cup breast and who after full consent understands and is prepared to accept all the potential risks and complications associated with implant-based reconstruction. These operations may also cost more than a standard mastectomy. Don't be afraid to ask your doctor about costs. It is your right to know.

Basically, what you are having with these new types of surgical approaches is a mastectomy—you still lose your entire breast, but you will lose less skin and sometimes the nipple and areola. Short-term results appear promising.

My rule of thumb is that if your breasts are on the larger side, aim to keep your breast if the area of DCIS can be removed with clear margins understanding that you will require radiation after your surgery. If your breast is on the smaller side and the area of DCIS is on the larger side, it is probably better to have a mastectomy. If your DCIS is within 1 to 2 cm of the nipple, the chance of the nipple being involved is high and removal of the nipple and, in my view, the areola is probably the safest approach if a mastectomy is planned.

CONTROL POINT #4 – WHAT WILL I DO ABOUT MY BREAST?

WARNING

Do not rush this decision! Once the breast is gone, it cannot be put back! Having a strong family history of breast cancer doesn't mean you need a mastectomy.

TIP

Understand the difference between a breast surgeon and a general surgeon. Breast surgeons know about the sentinel node biopsy technique and generally work in a team with oncologists. Your surgeon may also recommend oncoplastic surgery.

REMEMBER

If you want a mastectomy and feel more comfortable with a mastectomy rather than radiation treatment, go with your gut feeling. Understand the risks and benefits of keeping or losing your breast.

WHAT WILL I DO ABOUT MY ARMPIT?

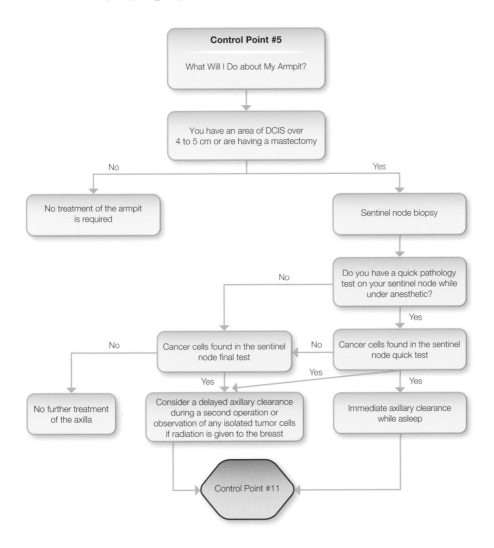

Control Point #5

What Will I Do about My Armpit?

↓

You have an area of DCIS over 4 to 5 cm or are having a mastectomy

No →

Yes →

No treatment of the armpit is required

Sentinel node biopsy

Do you have a quick pathology test on your sentinel node while under anesthetic?

No

Yes

Cancer cells found in the sentinel node final test

No

Cancer cells found in the sentinel node quick test

Yes

Yes

No

No further treatment of the axilla

Consider a delayed axillary clearance during a second operation or observation of any isolated tumor cells if radiation is given to the breast

Immediate axillary clearance while asleep

Control Point #11

5

Understanding the Lymphatic System Surrounding Your Breast

The second important preoperative decision is what to do about the armpit or **axilla**. DCIS on its own cannot spread to the armpit, but large areas of DCIS have a higher chance of unsuspected invasive cancer. You will recall, that in Table 1.1 (page 26), I showed you the results of a large study, where before surgery, 190 patients were thought to have DCIS using a core biopsy performed under a local anesthetic, whereas, after removal of the area using a general anesthetic, the abnormal area on the mammogram turned out to have areas of real or "invasive" cancer in almost one in five patients.

In most cases, for DCIS, you probably won't need anything done to your armpit unless your DCIS is on the larger side, perhaps over 4 or 5 cm, or your DCIS presents as a lump that you or your doctor can feel or if you choose to have a mastectomy. You will recall that earlier I likened the way that invasive breast cancer can spread to the idea of a rosebush in a garden patch, with the lymph glands in your armpit being in the adjacent garden patch.

The axilla is a pad of fat that contains lots of lymph glands, or "nodes." Lymph nodes are located in many parts of the body and are part of the immune system, which help us fight infections and cancer. For example, when you have a sore throat from the common cold, the lymph nodes are often tender and enlarged because the infection is being attacked and stopped by them. The same thing can happen if your DCIS progresses to invasive breast cancer.

The lymphatic system includes not only the lymph glands or "**lymph nodes**," but also a network of tiny channels connecting all the nodes called **lymph vessels**. The first draining lymph node from the involved breast is called the **sentinel node**, and it receives multiple lymphatic channels from the area in the breast where your DCIS first started. The sentinel node is a type of "guardian" lymph node, and it is thought that the lymphatic vessels drain there first before being connected by the lymph vessels to other lymph nodes. There are usually one to three sentinel nodes draining each breast.

Breast cancer can spread to the lymph nodes via the lymphatic system, and they are often the first port of call. Our lymph glands and our immune system are trying to stop the cancer from spreading any further. In many ways, the lymph nodes are like a filter trap in a sink. Figure 5.1 shows how the lymph glands are organized in the armpit around the pectoralis minor muscle, which is the muscle under the pectoralis major muscle. It is the pectoralis major that most people call "the pec," and it is prominent in weightlifters. Other lymph nodes are located above the collarbone (**supraclavicular fossa**) and beside the breastbone (**internal mammary chain**). These are often abbreviated by doctors as SCF or IMC lymph nodes.

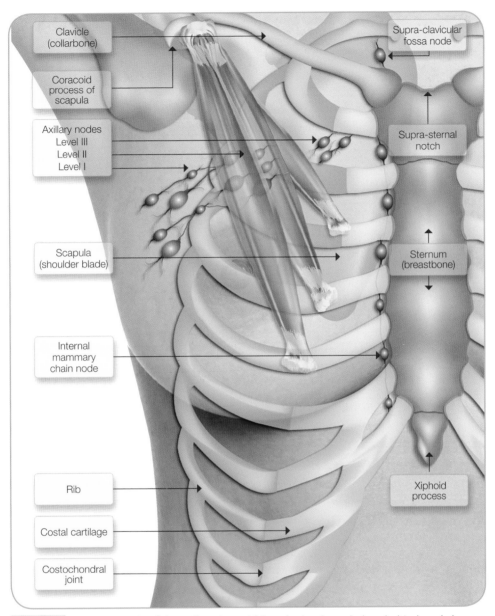

Clavicle
(collarbone)

Coracoid
process of
scapula

Axillary nodes
Level III
Level II
Level I

Scapula
(shoulder blade)

Internal
mammary
chain node

Rib

Costal cartilage

Costochondral
joint

Supra-clavicular
fossa node

Supra-sternal
notch

Sternum
(breastbone)

Xiphoid
process

Figure 5.1 The three levels of the axillary (armpit) lymph glands are below, behind, and above the pectoralis minor muscle, the small muscle behind the pectoralis major (not shown).

Deciding to Have a Sentinel Node Biopsy

These days, there are really only two choices for dealing with the lymph nodes if you have DCIS. The options are:

1. No sampling of the axillary lymph nodes (most common approach); Or . . .

2.   A sentinel node biopsy, where only the first node on the same side of the breast cancer is removed, and if that is clear, no further lymph nodes are taken.

Some surgeons, when they perform a mastectomy for a large area of DCIS may just take a sample of the lymph nodes in the axilla. Before the advent of the sentinel node technique, we used to advise a sample of the lower part of the Level I lymph nodes in the axilla. In the U.K., this is sometimes called a "4 node sample." In this technique, the aim is for the surgeon to remove at least four lymph nodes he or she can feel in the armpit starting at the point where the breast blends into the armpit region.

An "**axillary clearance**," where some or all of the lymph nodes from under the armpit are removed either during the mastectomy or breast conservation, is usually reserved for cases in which the sentinel node reveals cancer cells. In other words, it's performed only if your condition turns out to be cancer which has spread to the lymph nodes.

This can be a difficult concept to grasp, so I will go back to my garden example. Having a sentinel node mapping procedure and biopsy is a bit like finding a "runner" from the weed under the rosebush and following it into the next garden patch, then using a small spade to dig around the runner to see if it's taken root there as well. If the runner hasn't taken root and there are no weeds in the next garden patch, then removing some of the soil in that patch will not be necessary after examination with our small spade (sentinel node biopsy). If it has, then we will need a bigger spade to check the entire second patch and remove any weeds (axillary clearance). If there is cancer in the lymph nodes, then it is more than likely that somewhere surrounding the DCIS in your breast there are actual cancer cells that have broken through the duct, and it is now invasive cancer (Figure D on page 11).

The mapping procedure involves radioactive dye being injected around your DCIS, and over the next hour or two, it drains into the first filter trap or sentinel lymph node. This collection of radioactive dye in the sentinel node shows up on an X-ray taken using a **gamma camera**.

What Is the Chance That There Is Unsuspected Cancer within Your DCIS That Has Spread to the Lymph Glands?

Before I discuss the options for your armpit, it's very important to understand your own risk of cancer spreading from the breast to the armpit is usually very small. A landmark study from the University of California, San Francisco looked at the chance of having a cancerous lymph node involved in the armpit based on the size of the DCIS in the breast after careful examination following a mastectomy (Lagios 1982). Basically, the study found that the bigger the area of DCIS or the higher its grade, the higher the risk of cancer spreading through the duct (this is sometimes called "microinvasion" or "occult invasion") to the armpit. For women who had an area of DCIS over 50 mm as measured by the pathologist, the incidence of "occult invasion" occurred in about seven out of ten patients (69%), and the chance of the disease being in the axillary lymph nodes was about 8 in 100 (7.7%). If the DCIS was under 50 mm in size, then the incidence of lymph node involvement in the axilla was zero.

Before sentinel node procedures, I used this data to recommend a "low **axillary dissection**" for my patients with areas of DCIS that were over 50 mm based on the Lagios data. Today, because the sentinel node technique has far less complications, I never recommend an axillary dissection but always push for a sentinel node biopsy if you have "high-risk" DCIS, which I will define for you below.

A research paper examined twenty-two publications which studied over 3,000 patients on the likelihood of a sentinel node being positive if you have DCIS using a technique called a **meta-analysis** (Ansari et al. 2008). They found that the incidence of a sentinel node being involved was about 7% if performed before surgery but lower and potentially less reliable at 4% if the sentinel node biopsy was done after the DCIS was already surgically excised.

Ansari found the following features predicted a higher chance of a real or invasive breast cancer after surgical removal of the presumed DCIS and represented "high-risk" lesions:

- a palpable lump
- a lump visible on your mammogram or ultrasound
- a high-grade lesion or
- a large area of DCIS size (usually at least 4 cm).

For a large area of DCIS it is often difficult for the pathologist to examine every single piece of it. Usually representative "sections" are taken from the abnormal area. Sentinel node biopsy in high-risk patients with DCIS can therefore be a back-up mechanism to discover unsuspected areas of invasion that have already spread to the lymph node.

If abnormal cells are found in a lymph node and you only have DCIS, we sometimes ask the pathologist to go back and have a second look and even take more, usually deeper, sections of the DCIS in the breast. Sometimes, they find an abnormal area of "microinvasion" in these deeper sections, other times they only find more DCIS.

How Is a Sentinel Node Biopsy Done?

For a sentinel node procedure to be successful, you need a good team of doctors who work well together. You need a radiologist to inject the radioactive dye and read the subsequent X-rays, and usually the surgeon will inject a blue dye around the cancer while you're anesthetized. That dye can be taken up by the lymphatics and drain to the sentinel node. You also need a surgeon who has the right equipment, including a probe like a Geiger counter that can detect the radiation in the sentinel node. The sentinel node is found, or "mapped," using up to three techniques. These are:

1. a nuclear medicine test called **lymphoscintigraphy** (lymphatic mapping) that's performed before the operation

2. a blue dye test, also performed by the surgeon as part of the operation

3. a scan using a handheld probe performed by the surgeon during surgery.

Although surgeons often perform a "quick-test" on the sentinel node for patients with invasive breast cancer while they are under anesthetic, I am not so sure it is all that useful if you have DCIS. Most women with DCIS do not have a positive sentinel node. If it is involved, it is often only tiny and would be easily missed by a quick test such as a **frozen section**, a procedure in which the pathologist urgently cuts the sentinel node in half and swipes it across a slide (a bit like a Pap smear slide) and looks for cancer cells.

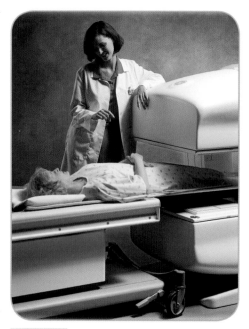

Figure 5.2 A gamma camera, which picks up the low-dose radiation emitted from your sentinel node.

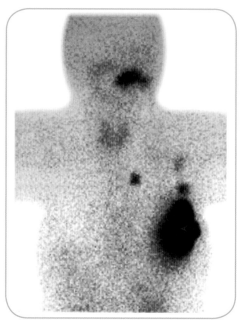

Figure 5.3 A sentinel node scan done before surgery, showing uptake behind the breastbone, in the armpit, and around the breast tumor.

Lymphoscintigraphy (Lymphatic Mapping)

Typically, a tiny amount of a radiation-labeled material called a colloid is injected above or around the tumor, or sometimes around the nipple. The radioactive materials, trapped by the draining sentinel lymph nodes, are seen with a special X-ray machine called a gamma camera (Figure 5.2) as "hot spots" one or two hours after the injection of the colloid (Figure 5.3). These nodes are then often marked on the skin with a waterproof marker to help the surgeon know where to make his cut and start looking for the gland.

Don't be frightened about this test. It uses very low-dose radiation. Your doctors will usually use a local anesthetic before injecting the dye (and maybe you should insist on it). And remember that just because you're mapping the sentinel nodes doesn't mean that the cancer has spread to them. It just lets your surgeon find the spot where it's most likely for any unsuspected cancer within your DCIS to spread first.

Blue Dye

Intra-operative blue dye may be injected during the operation and taken up by lymphatic channels and nodes, allowing your surgeon a second way to see the sentinel node (the first is the Geiger counter probe). Don't worry, you won't feel the needle at all. A combination technique is ideal but don't worry too much if they use one technique over another. It really depends on the expertise and the resources the surgeon possesses.

Handheld Probe

This is a type of Geiger counter used to find the sentinel nodes that the nuclear physician has marked on the skin and that are shown in the X-ray above (Figure 5.4). Usually, the surgeon double-checks the area, because sometimes sentinel nodes are "hot," as shown by the probe, but were not visible on the X-ray, usually because of technical reasons.

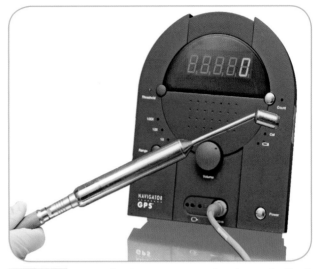

Figure 5.4 A type of Geiger counter used to detect the "hot" sentinel nodes during surgery.

Sentinel Node Pathology Testing

The sentinel node is usually cut up into about six pieces and the pathologist examines it carefully during the week after your surgery. In addition, the naked eye does not see all of these small cells, which are often smaller than a grain of sand. We need to use a special stain called an **immunohistochemistry (IHC) stain**, which can sometimes show the cancer cells as black or dark brown or red.

Figure 5.5 is an example of a sentinel node as seen by a pathologist under a microscope. The purple section is unstained by immunohistochemistry and shows no visible cancer cells, but on the right side, with the IHC stain added, there are some red cells visible—these are cancer cells.

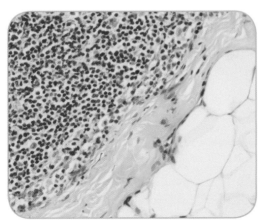 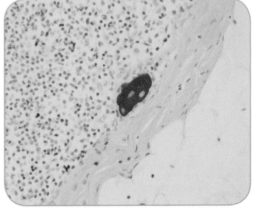

Figure 5.5 A sentinel node as seen with the naked eye (left), and with special immunohistochemical (IHC) stain (the brown spots on the right are called micrometastases).

What Happens If I Have Cancer Cells in My Sentinel Lymph Node?

First of all, don't panic. The consequences of small deposits of cells in the sentinel lymph node even in invasive breast cancer is still hotly debated.

A number of questions arise. Firstly, are the cells in the sentinel node a false-positive finding related to cells being dislodged at the time of your original core biopsy or at the time of your surgery? Or...

Is the growth in the sentinel node real and reflecting a small cancer that has spread in the lymphatics and could spread elsewhere if not treated with hormonal treatment or chemotherapy?

There is a lot of controversy about what tiny deposits of cancer cells in a sentinel node really mean when found by an immunohistochemistry (IHC) stain. A lot of research has been done as to whether small deposits called **micrometastases** or micromets, or even smaller deposits called **isolated tumor cells** or "ITCs," impact a patient's prognosis.

The international classification committee has tried to differentiate "minor" spread to the armpit, or isolated tumor cells (ITCs), from micrometastases primarily on the basis of size. ITCs are defined as single cells or small clusters of cells not greater than 0.2 mm in largest dimension and are classified as pN0(i). Micrometastases are defined as tumor deposits greater than 0.2 mm, but not greater than 2.0 mm in largest dimension. Cases in which only micro-metastases are detected (i.e., not greater than 2 mm) are classified pN1mi. Where cancer is greater than 2 mm, this is called a **macrometastasis**.

The problem is that most of the research has been done for patients with invasive breast cancer and not DCIS. A small study from the Netherlands was performed, however, in sixty-six patients with pure DCIS treated years earlier who had at least five lymph glands removed. The researchers went back and performed the IHC or immunohistochemistry test on these lymph nodes. They found that, in retrospect, seven of the original sixty-six patients (11%) had cells in the lymph node of which six were ITCs and one was a micromet. After an average follow-up period of over seven years, all patients remained disease-free without chemotherapy or hormonal treatment (Broekhuizen et al. 2006).

It is, therefore, fair to say that the management of patients with apparently pure DCIS in the breast and some cells in the sentinel node remains contentious.

So what can we make of all this. It's certainly confusing. Here are my thoughts until new evidence emerges:

- For patients with "high-risk" DCIS, as defined above, who have a chance of having unsuspected microinvasive disease, a sentinel node biopsy should be considered in an attempt to avoid a second anesthetic.

- Patients with DCIS having a mastectomy or a large excision close to the axilla, or breast reconstruction involving the axilla, should also be considered for a sentinel node biopsy as they could be found to have invasive disease. The procedure is usually impossible or much harder to do later.

- The sentinel node biopsy is not a perfect test, and sometimes the results are "clear" or "negative"; but if a full dissection were done, we would find cancer left behind in another (non-sentinel) node, and hence it's called "false negative." The main reason a sentinel node biopsy is done is to avoid the higher complication rates that come with a full axillary clearance, such as pins and needles over the inner upper aspect of your arm and swelling of the arm, called lymphedema.

- Don't worry too much if all you have is ITCs in the sentinel node. These may simply be "visitors" and harmless, rather than "residents," which can lodge and start growing. Just because a cell is dislodged doesn't mean it's dangerous. Just because a pea falls into your kitchen sink and gets caught, doesn't mean it's going to grow there.

- If the sentinel node biopsy shows a micromet, radiation to the breast (which treats the lower part of the axillary lymph nodes) will almost certainly control the situation. If you are in this situation and you have had a mastectomy, it is likely that the only gland involved is the sentinel node and a case could be made for just examining your armpit at regular intervals rather than going back and having a full axillary dissection. If you're the type of personality who wants more certainty, going back and doing an axillary sample or a dissection only of level one of the axilla would be reasonable.

- If the sentinel node shows a "macrometastasis," meaning that the cancer in your sentinel node is greater than 2 mm and has probably been there for some time, I would lean towards an axillary dissection and additional hormonal treatment or chemotherapy depending on your age and general health as you really have invasive breast cancer mixed in with your DCIS.

Side Effects of a Sentinel Node Biopsy

The blue dye may turn your urine blue-green for about twenty-four hours. The blue dye is sometimes confused as a bruise, which can also occur after surgery. The skin over your breast may be stained blue for three to four weeks, but this is rarely permanent (Figure 5.6). Mild allergic reactions can occur in 1 to 2% of patients. Severe allergic reactions are extremely rare. If this occurs, it usually causes no serious problems because your anesthetist is watching closely over you. Infection is always a possibility with any surgery. If this occurs, your scar may be red and hot, and you may have a temperature. Call your doctor or breast care nurse if this occurs.

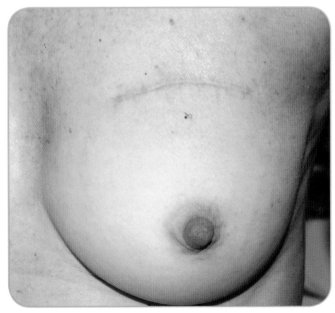

Figure 5.6 Blue stain on the skin after a Patent Blue injection may take several days or weeks to resolve and may be confused with a bruise.

Lymphedema is swelling of the arm that occurs after axillary treatment of any sort. The risk is estimated to be 1 to 2% after a sentinel node biopsy. Lymphedema of the arm is an accumulation of lymph fluid in the tissues of your arm, which causes swelling. Having surgery under your armpit increases the risk of scarring and what we call back-pressure. It's a bit like the difference between a fast-flowing river and a slow-flowing river that is blocked by rocks. The one blocked by rocks backs up and the water is often murkier than a fast-flowing river. Edema can also occur in your breast if it has been conserved, and this is discussed further in "Control Point #16 – Do I Need Radiation Therapy?"

Common early symptoms of lymphedema include heaviness, aching, and/or fluctuating swelling in the hands or fingers, or tightening of your rings. Later symptoms include swelling of the forearm or upper arm or the whole arm. These symptoms may initially settle overnight, but when more advanced, they can become permanent. An important goal is to keep your arm feeling soft with regular moisturizers to avoid fibrosis (hardness) from developing.

Technologies such as bioimpedance can detect early changes of fluid at a cellular level up to ten months earlier than detection with a tape measure. If you are worried about your arm, an L-Dex® measurement may be useful. See http://international.l-dex.com/what-is-l-dex. Taking control means feeling empowered to manage your own symptoms according to your lifestyle. Exercise and movement are strongly recommended because muscle contraction helps to push the lymph fluid through the lymphatic channels, reducing the chance of swelling. Some good information is available from the National Cancer Institute Web site, www.cancer.gov/cancertopics/pdq/supportivecare/lymphedema or from the Westmead Breast Cancer Institute Web site, www.bci.org.au/about-breast-cancer/fact-sheets/183-lymphoedema.html.

A really simple but important step in preventing infection after lymphedema is to ensure your skin does not become dry or irritated by using a moisturizer, one that does not contain perfume. Massaging the arm daily in an upward direction assists the fluid in moving upward rather than staying in the arm. The lymphatics do not have a pump or one-way valves like your arteries, so rely on gentle massage and exercise to assist the movement and drainage of lymph fluid.

The bottom line is that most women with DCIS don't get lymphedema.

CONTROL POINT #5 – WHAT WILL I DO ABOUT MY ARMPIT?

WARNING

A sentinel node biopsy should be considered if you have "high-risk" DCIS such as a large area (over 4–5 cm), or if your DCIS first presents as a lump. An axillary dissection is not recommended.

TIP

Moisturize your arm regularly after surgery, all the way up to your armpit, if you have had a sentinel node biopsy.

REMEMBER

Talk to your surgeon about the advantages and disadvantages of a sentinel node biopsy versus just watching your armpit. Usually we do not operate on the armpit for DCIS. Don't rush this decision.

IF I HAVE A MASTECTOMY, CAN I WEAR AN EXTERNAL PROSTHESIS?

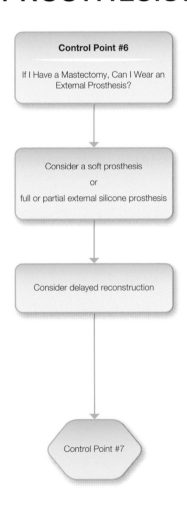

Control Point #6

If I Have a Mastectomy, Can I Wear an External Prosthesis?

Consider a soft prosthesis
or
full or partial external silicone prosthesis

Consider delayed reconstruction

Control Point #7

6

If I Have a Mastectomy, Can I Wear an External Prosthesis?

If you don't have a reconstruction, getting an external **breast prosthesis** is a good idea. This can be challenging at times and depends on how much support and information you get after your operation. The best people to talk to about a prosthesis are your discharge planner, social worker, or breast care nurse. Wearing an external prosthesis may help with your balance, symmetry, self-esteem, and confidence.

What Is a Breast Prosthesis?

A breast prosthesis is essentially an external, artificial breast shape or mound worn inside your bra or swimsuit. It's sometimes referred to as an external breast form. It is not an internal breast prosthesis or implant which I will discuss in the next Control Point. Many women feel quite self-conscious after a mastectomy because they may appear lopsided in clothes. A prosthesis can be temporary (usually lightweight) or permanent (weighted or lightweight), and some are suitable for active sports including swimming. All breast prostheses come in various skin tones and may be made from silicone or lighter materials.

What Types of Breast Prostheses Are Available?

You'll probably want to buy two types of breast prostheses: a non-weighted and a weighted one. A non-weighted foam or polyfill form is recommended when you're first recovering from surgery because it's softer and most comfortable over your healing skin (Figure 6.1).

Soft prostheses are also useful for informal leisure activities and feel good during warm weather and while swimming. They're conveniently machine washable and lightweight. In different countries they may be called "comfies," "softies," "falsies," or "filler." You may find that the soft-form prosthesis can "ride up" because it's so light. It may look better if you adjust the stuffing and pin it to the bottom of your bra cup. If you want to wear a bra with your soft prosthesis, try one that is soft and stretchy, without an underwire. Remember, your first bra after a mastectomy has to be easy to take on and off because your shoulder may be stiff at first if you have had surgery on your lymph glands.

Weighted silicone prostheses are still very soft but add the weight and balance that you need to reduce the potential for neck and back problems. They are hand washable and look and feel better than soft prostheses because they're fitted to match the size, weight, and shape of your own breast. These too are worn externally. The added weight of a silicone prosthesis usually allows it to sit more easily at the same level as your other breast. If a silicone prosthesis "rides up," it might not be heavy enough.

After breast surgery, and also after radiation therapy, your chest area can be extra sensitive, so it's best to delay getting a silicone prosthesis until your chest area is fully healed after surgery, which generally takes about eight weeks. If you are having radiation treatment to the chest wall, wait at least six to eight weeks after it's completed and any skin reaction has settled.

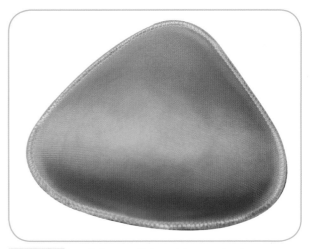

Figure 6.1 A soft-form or lightweight prosthesis.

You might want to ask your fitting service for a reassessment if you're not happy with how your prosthesis fits you. You really need to talk to your team about the style of your prosthesis, but the options include:

- Asymmetrical prostheses, often called classic style. One designed only for the left side and one only for the right side extend into the armpit (Figure 6.2, right).

- Symmetrical prostheses include the "pear shape" (also known as teardrop or oval prosthesis) or the "triangle shape." The pear shape prostheses work on either side and can be worn sideways filling the area towards your arm, or straight up for center fullness and cleavage. Triangles, which are very popular, have been on the market since the early to mid-1990s and come in a large variety of shapes, skin tones, and weights that allow the fit to be more customized to your body shape and size (Figure 6.2, left).

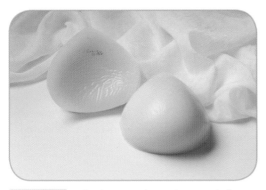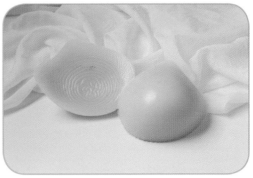

Figure 6.2 Soft silicone gel prostheses—left, triangle (symmetrical) and right, classical (asymmetrical).

A silicone prosthesis can be heavy, especially for larger-breasted women, and you may find it tiring. But the balanced weight it provides helps to keep your shoulders even and your posture straight. This makes it easier on your neck and shoulder.

Prices for silicone prostheses range from under $100 to about $500 for high-quality products. For public (uninsured) patients in Australia and the U.K., prostheses are free, at least for the first one. In the U.S., some states mandate that insurance companies need to provide at least some reimbursement. Check with your insurer or government program to learn what help is available to you. Many private insurance companies pay for a breast prosthesis and a bra. In the U.S., Medicare will not pay for any bra unless it has a built-in pocket produced by the manufacturer. Medicare allows one silicone breast prosthesis form every two years based on medical necessity. Six mastectomy bras every year are also usually allowed. Medicare usually pays for a camisole immediately following surgery, and one light-weight form every six months is normally covered. Medicare rebates may vary in different U.S. states so please check with the local social security office.

In Australia, an external prosthesis is reimbursable up to AUD$800 every two years for two sides or AUD$400 for one side. For more information see www.humanservices.gov.au/customer/services/medicare/external-breast-prostheses-reimbursement-program.

There are also special smaller prostheses for women who have had breast conservation surgery. These may be worn inside the bra and are shaped to fill out a small part of the breast (Figure 6.3). They are made of the same silicone material as most full-breast prostheses. Some have a stick-on backing.

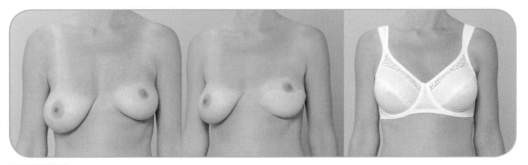

Figure 6.3 A smaller partial prosthesis, sometimes useful after breast conservation.

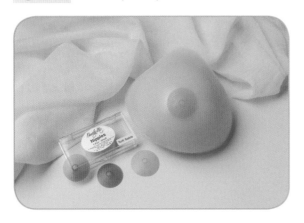

Nipples can be added to prostheses if required (Figure 6.4). Swimsuits and lingerie designed for women who have had mastectomies are available by catalog from Lands' End, Sears, Nordstrom, and J.C. Penney in the U.S.; Myer and David Jones in Australia; and in small shops and department stores in several countries.

Figure 6.4 An example of a breast prosthesis with optional stick-on nipple.

The clothing comes with a pocket to hold the prosthesis. You can also have pockets sewn into the bras or swimsuits you already own. You should be able to wear a normal bra with a prosthesis. The bra should fit well and offer medium to firm control. You could get a pocket sewn into your bra or sew two ribbons across the inside to hold the prosthesis. Wearing a soft cotton bra that opens at the front with a soft-form prosthesis is a good way to start, particularly if your arm is restricted after surgery to the armpit (Figure 6.5).

These bras, available from most major manufacturers who specialize in post–breast surgery products, have pockets in both cups to fit a soft-form prosthesis. The soft cotton helps with any discomfort associated with your scar. They are also very good during radiotherapy not only because you can get them off quickly for your daily treatment but also because these bras are relatively inexpensive so it's no problem if you get any of the skin marks from your radiotherapy on the bra.

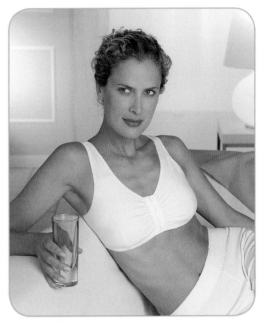

Figure 6.5 Front-closing cotton bras with pockets are best just after your surgery and during radiotherapy.

There are also some very practical and attractive bras and swimwear that are designed to hold a prosthesis (Figures 6.6 and 6.7). Make sure you get an appointment for a fitting for your prosthesis. Don't be rushed into making your choice. Look at and try on as many as possible and be sure that the one you buy comes with a 12-month warranty. When you go for a fitting, take a shirt, blouse, and/or T-shirt so that you can see the final result.

Check that the prosthesis fills your bra cup at both the top and the bottom. A softer silicone prosthesis will give a more natural shape. Stand upright and check in the mirror for shape and a good match to your natural breast. Swing your arms back and forth to check that the form is not too full under your arm.

Care of Your Prosthesis

Most prostheses, properly cared for, last two to three years. Ensure that you:

- hand wash your prosthesis regularly, preferably daily
- store the prosthesis in the box it came in to help it keep its shape
- avoid wearing a silicone-filled prosthesis in a saltwater or chlorinated pool or in a heated sauna or spa, as it may heat up against your skin.

The Ideal Bra after a Mastectomy

The Breast Cancer Care organization in the U.K. has published some excellent guidelines called "A Confident Choice: Breast Prostheses, Bras and Clothes after Surgery." Their advice states that a proper bra should have:

- good separation between the cups, which should not be too low

- good depth under the arm with a lower cut to avoid rubbing and an underband (below cups) at least 10 mm deep

- a firm or elasticized upper edge to the cups and good straps

- full cups to cover the prosthesis

- at least two hooks to fasten at the back (more in larger sizes).

Also look for a bra that is wider under the arm so there is greater support around the back and to cover any scars or areas of puckering around your scar. Most of these features can be seen below and can be found at their Web site, www.breastcancercare.org.uk.

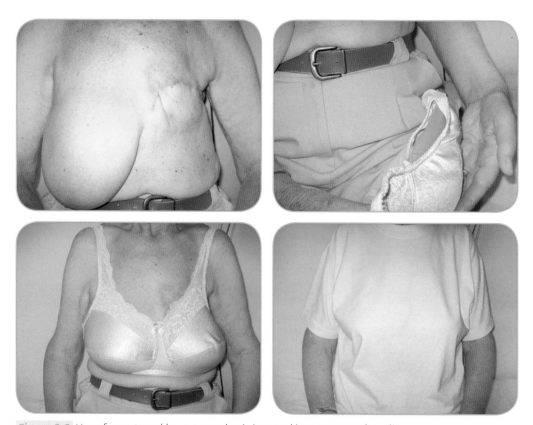

Figure 6.6 Use of an external breast prosthesis inserted into a custom bra slip.

At first, it's a good idea to buy just one bra (or at most two), in case it turns out to be unsuitable—for example, if it's not comfortable or the cup doesn't cover the prosthesis well enough, or in case your bra size changes with changes in your weight as a result of your treatment. You could keep the bra in its packaging until you have your prosthesis fitting so that you can change it if you need to. It's advisable to purchase three bras at a time (one in the wash, one to wear, and one as a spare). Also, it is highly recommended that you go back to your fitter every six months, since if you gain or lose weight, it will change the look and weight of the remaining natural breast and therefore how the prosthesis fits and mimics your body.

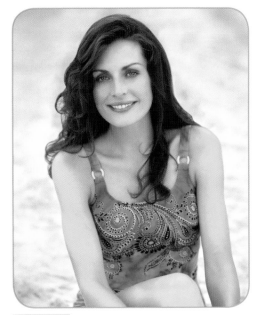

Figure 6.7 Specialized swimwear with adjustable shoulder straps and a special bust with pockets to insert a breast prosthesis.

CONTROL POINT #6 – IF I HAVE A MASTECTOMY, CAN I WEAR AN EXTERNAL PROSTHESIS?

WARNING

After breast surgery your chest area can be extra sensitive, so it's best to delay getting an external silicone prosthesis until about eight weeks after your surgery and/or radiation therapy is completed.

TIP

Wearing a soft cotton bra that opens at the front with a soft-form prosthesis is a good way to start after your surgery, particularly if your arm is restricted after surgery to the armpit or you are having radiation therapy.

REMEMBER

Talk to your bra and prosthesis fitter or breast care nurse about your options for a bra or prosthesis sooner rather than later after your surgery.

IF I HAVE A MASTECTOMY, WHAT ARE MY OPTIONS FOR BREAST RECONSTRUCTION?

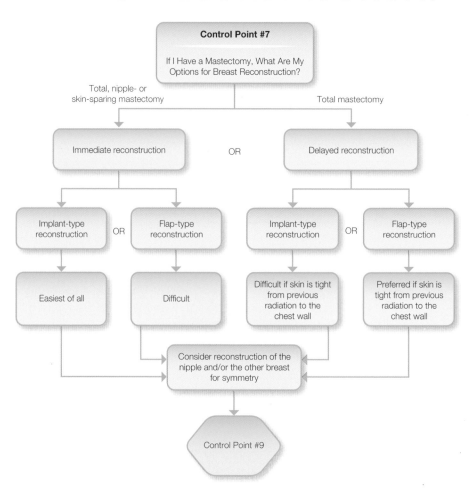

If I Have a Mastectomy, What Are My Options for Breast Reconstruction?

Having a breast reconstruction is a very personal decision and you should not be pressured one way or another by your partner, friends, or doctors. Take control of this decision by getting as much information as you can from your treating doctors, support groups, organizations, and if possible, other women who have gone through the same procedure.

Don't feel rushed by your surgeon's operating schedule; take the time to work out the best option for you right now if you are having a mastectomy for your DCIS. Because DCIS is not cancer, you have a very good prognosis and your treatment, if it remains pure DCIS after your final pathology report is back, will mainly consist of your surgery. It makes sense, therefore, to consider having a reconstruction immediately given cure rates after a mastectomy are close to 100%.

Your options include: never having a reconstruction for your DCIS; having it done in a few years (**delayed reconstruction**); or having it done at the same time as your mastectomy (**immediate reconstruction**). If you're having an immediate reconstruction, the plastic surgeon will usually take over directly after the mastectomy, while you're still under anesthetic. As mentioned earlier, some surgeons are trained to do both the mastectomy and a more limited type of reconstruction that is often referred to as oncoplastic surgery.

There are many myths about having a breast reconstruction after a mastectomy, but one thing that's certain is that it's a complex decision. Factors that influence this decision include not only your thoughts and feelings, but also the availability of expertise and resources, such as your specialist team and the availability of operating theater time.

What Is Breast Reconstruction?

Breast reconstruction is a complex procedure, and often, you may need two or more operations to achieve a correctly positioned new breast after a mastectomy for your DCIS. In the past, the mastectomy was called a "**total mastectomy**" as it removed the entire breast and nipple region and a lot of the skin of your breast. A mastectomy without a reconstruction essentially means you have a flat chest wall as shown in Figure 4.5 on page 63. This meant that there wasn't a lot of skin tissue to use which either had to be stretched with an expander (see Figure 7.1) or by moving skin (and muscle) from another part of your body.

More recently, surgeons have begun to preserve more of your skin. I discussed the role of skin-sparing mastectomy (which involves keeping more skin but removing the nipple and areola) or nipple-sparing mastectomy (where a lot more of the skin envelope and its natural contour, including the nipple and areola, is preserved and filled with an implant or a muscle flap) in "Control Point #4 – What Will I Do about My Breast?" This chapter deals with how to fill the gap that is left once all your breast is removed with a nipple-sparing, skin-sparing, or standard mastectomy.

Whatever reconstructive procedure you choose, your breasts probably won't be completely symmetrical afterward and will never be like your own natural breast. Still, many women choose to have reconstructions. Different approaches to breast reconstruction include:

- using tissue expanders and breast implants
- using your body's own tissue ("tissue" or "flap" reconstruction)
- using a combination of tissue reconstruction and implants.

Understand what breast reconstruction surgery can do for you, but also be aware of what it won't do for you. It will involve more surgery that takes longer under the anesthetic than surgery without a reconstruction. It is associated with more side effects, but it will give you a "mound," either constructed from your own tissue or using a silicone implant.

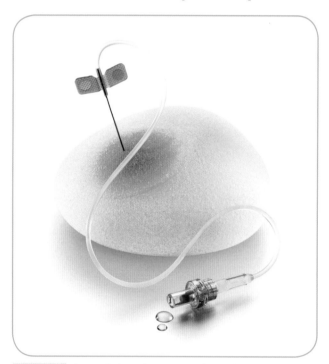

Figure 7.1 Pictured above is an expander, to be inserted behind the pectoralis major muscle. Salt water (saline) is injected into its magnetic port (at tip of green butterfly needle) once a week for roughly four to six weeks.

The breast reconstruction process can also include reconstruction of your nipple, but some women omit this step because the reconstructed nipple is only cosmetic and will not function like your natural nipple. If your nipple is preserved as part of a nipple-sparing mastectomy, it will almost certainly have no sensation or markedly reduced sensation.

Finally, you may choose to have surgery on your other breast, even if it's healthy, so that it more closely matches the shape and size of your reconstructed breast. This can, for example, involve an enhancement, or more usually a "lift" (mastopexy) or a reduction, particularly if you had large breasts to start with. As discussed in "Control Point #4 – What Will I Do about My Breast?," a mastectomy with or without a reconstruction may be discussed for your normal side, particularly if you have a very strong family history.

When Can I Have Breast Reconstruction?

If you think you may want a breast reconstruction, it's very important to discuss this before your operation. Ask your breast surgeon to arrange an appointment with a plastic surgeon before your mastectomy to discuss whether or not you are more suited to an immediate reconstruction, a delayed reconstruction, or no reconstruction. It is becoming more common for breast surgeons to now do their own reconstructions, particularly the less complicated types of reconstructions not involving flap surgery.

You may want to see one or two reconstructive surgeons who work with your breast surgeon. It may be best to see one who has experience in all types of reconstructions, including implants and non-implant procedures using your own tissue. Ask to see some photographs of their work, or better still, see if you can talk to one or two of their previous patients.

Ultimately, your own feelings, thoughts, and instincts are critical. Take control here and don't be rushed. It may take a few extra days to get all the information you need.

Different Types of Breast Reconstruction

Tissue Expansion and Breast Implants

A breast implant is a round or teardrop-shaped silicone shell that's filled with salt water (saline) or silicone gel. A plastic surgeon places the implant behind the muscle in your chest (pectoral muscle) in a manner similar to that which occurs during breast augmentation (enlargement) surgery (Figure 7.1). Sometimes, a mastectomy is done on both sides and bilateral implants are inserted, particularly if there is a strong family history of breast cancer.

Most women require a two-stage process, using a temporary tissue expander before the permanent implant is placed. Tissue expansion involves stretching your remaining chest skin and soft tissues to make room for the breast implant. After the tissue expander is implanted, you'll need to visit your doctor's office every week or two, for a total of five or six visits, to have small amounts of salt water inserted into the expander through a magnetic port. The port is magnetic so that the nurse or doctor can use a magnet to quickly find the access port and inject the saline. It's a bit like a beach balloon that slowly gets inflated with saline rather than air (Figure 7.2).

The skin is stretched slowly to avoid too much discomfort or pressure as the implant expands, but some minor discomfort is often associated with the procedure (Figure 7.3). The first day or so after your surgery is usually when you'll be the most uncomfortable.

After the tissue expansion process is complete, your surgeon will perform further surgery to remove the expander and replace it with a permanent implant, which has a more natural look and feel. This normally takes place six to nine months after the implant is first inserted. Once complete, the final result can look very good in a bra (Figure 7.4). Over time, implants may leak or need replacement, but usually not for eight to ten years or more. However, implants involve less surgery, less pain, shorter recovery, no additional scar, and less expense than **flap reconstruction**.

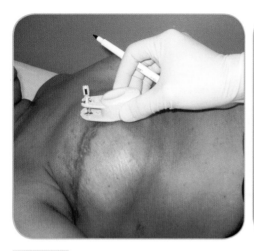
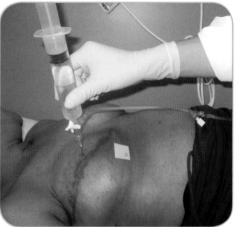

Figure 7.2 This woman had a mastectomy and a sub-pectoral implant. A magnet (left) is used to find the exact location of the port under the skin. A needle and syringe full of saline (right) is then used to inflate the implant at regular intervals.

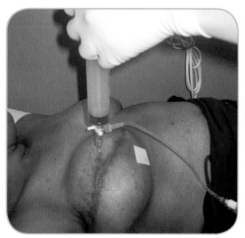
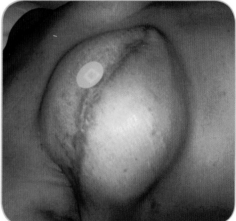

Figure 7.3 An additional 50 mL of saline was inserted into the implant before the patient's radiation treatment started.

Some women are able to go through a one-stage implantation process—receiving the final, permanent implant at the time of the mastectomy. This is only possible if more of the skin is preserved with a skin-sparing mastectomy or skin, nipple and areola in a nipple-sparing mastectomy (see Figure 4.10 on page 66). These one-step procedures allow more room for an immediate silicone implant, thus avoiding the expander, the multiple visits to inflate it with saline, and a second procedure months later to replace the temporary expander with a permanent implant.

If you have a skin-sparing or nipple-sparing mastectomy, the surgeon removes the DCIS and the remainder of the breast through a small incision usually around the areola area of the nipple. The surgeon leaves most of the breast skin, creating a natural skin envelope, or pocket, that is filled with

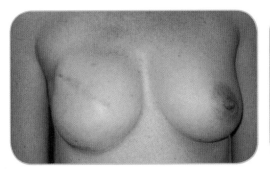 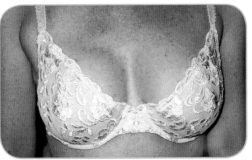

Figure 7.4 A mound has been produced that looks good in a bra.

a breast implant or with your own tissue from another part of your body. The main difference with a traditional mastectomy is that it removes very little skin, which can then be filled immediately rather than waiting for the stretching procedure shown in Figures 7.2 and 7.3.

Although an implant reconstruction may be performed at the same time as your mastectomy, or at a later time, it cannot usually be performed after radiation therapy is given to the chest area after a mastectomy (**postmastectomy radiation therapy**). This is because radiation treatment can cause tightening and reduced flexibility or stretch of the skin, making the implant impossible to insert.

Sometimes, though, it can be done if there is some stretch left in the skin. If radiation therapy is necessary, a flap reconstruction is preferable if a delayed reconstruction is done because the irradiated skin can be removed and replaced with healthy skin from another part of the body ("**donor site**"). But don't get too concerned, as the chance of you needing radiation therapy after a mastectomy for DCIS is probably less than 1 or 2 in 100. As I will show in "Control Point #16 – Do I Need Radiation Therapy?," radiation after a mastectomy is possibly indicated if the surgical margins close to your chest wall are very close or involved.

Tissue or Flap Reconstruction

This is the most complex reconstructive option, but it has the advantage of a more natural look and feel after a mastectomy for your DCIS. With tissue or flap reconstruction, your surgeon moves a section of skin, muscle, fat, and blood vessels from one part of your body to your chest to create a new breast mound. The nipple can be recreated later. Flap reconstructions require three to eight hours of surgery, and sometimes longer.

Because muscle flap reconstruction requires healthy blood vessels, women with diabetes, connective tissue disease, vascular disease, previous major abdominal surgery, or a history of smoking may need to consider other options. During a flap reconstruction, flaps of muscle and skin are taken from the back, abdomen, or buttocks. In some cases, the skin and tissue need to be expanded further with a breast implant to achieve the desired breast size.

Flaps can be "free" or "attached" from the donor source and original blood supply. A **free flap** means that the "flap" of skin, fat, and muscle tissue is completely detached and then connected to a new supply of blood vessels in the original breast area without tunneling under the skin. The surgeon detaches the tissue completely from its blood supply and uses microsurgery to reattach the tissue flap to new blood vessels near your chest. Because of the intricate nature of reattaching blood vessels using microsurgery, free flap surgery typically takes longer to complete than **pedicle flap** (attached flap) surgery does.

Not all plastic surgeons can do microsurgery. The free flap procedure can have a higher complication rate, so make sure that you see a highly skilled specialist. However, many surgeons believe that the free flap allows them to create a more natural shape than the pedicle flap. A pedicle flap is tunneled under the skin whilst the flap is connected to the original donor source and blood supply. There are four common types of flap reconstructions: latissimus dorsi, TRAM, DIEP, and gluteal.

The latissimus dorsi muscle (LD) flap is taken from the back, with its own blood supply, and is tunneled under the skin to the front of the chest (Figure 7.5). The flap is not large, and it may therefore be necessary to use a small implant as well as the flap. This is a useful technique if you do not have large breasts or if previous abdominal surgery prevents using abdominal tissue.

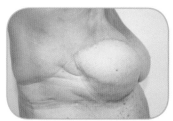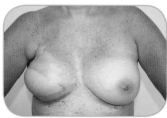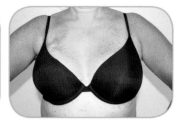

Figure 7.5 Different views of a latissimus dorsi muscle flap. A sub-pectoral implant was also inserted on the left side to match the size of the new breast on the right side.

The **transverse rectus abdominus muscle (TRAM) flap** procedure uses tissue tunneled from your lower abdomen—including a full thickness of skin, fat, and muscle—that is either attached to its own blood supply (pedicle) or detached (free) from its own blood supply. This muscle flap will create a reconstructed breast at the mastectomy site with no areola or nipple (Figure 7.7). It also means that some of the fat and muscle in your abdomen is used, so a "tummy tuck" is an added bonus. The downside is that there can be more weakness in the abdomen, and a hernia is a possible complication. There is no doubt that this is a major procedure, and it can take many weeks to fully recover, but most women are happy with the very natural feel of their new breast. Although the scars after a TRAM look prominent at first, they will fade and be less visible within four to six months of surgery.

The **deep inferior epigastric perforator (DIEP) flap** abdominal procedure uses blood vessels in the abdomen that travel through (perforate) the rectus abdominus muscle to supply the overlying abdominal skin. This newer procedure is almost the same as a TRAM flap, but skin and fat are the only tissues removed, so no muscle is taken. The flap uses a free (detached) flap approach, which allows you to retain more strength in your abdomen. If your surgeon can't perform a DIEP flap procedure for anatomical reasons, he or she might opt instead for the muscle-sparing free

TRAM flap. Studies have shown that there are fewer abdominal complications from the DIEP flap because muscle is not taken. The **superficial inferior epigastric artery (SIEA) flap** is very similar but uses different blood vessels. The **thoracodorsal artery perforator flap (TAP flap)** is also similar to the latissimus dorsi muscle (LD) flap but doesn't use the underlying muscle. A good Web site for more information is www.microsurgeon.org. The **gluteal (or buttock) flap** is a free flap procedure that takes tissue—possibly including muscle—from your buttocks and transplants it to your chest area after the mastectomy is finished.

Antibiotics are often given before and after surgery to reduce the risk of infection. Table 7.1 summarizes the different types of flap reconstructions. The British Association of Plastic, Reconstructive and Aesthetic Surgeons (BAPRAS) is also useful, see their Web site www.bapras.org.uk.

Not all women choose to have nipple reconstruction. It's entirely up to you. Some women can't really be bothered going back for surgery and it's perfectly okay if you feel that way. The nipple can also be reconstructed and tattooed to reproduce an appropriate color to match with your other breast. The reconstructed nipple will not have sensation. Silicone "stick-on" nipples are also available.

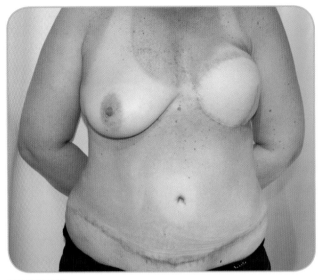

Figure 7.6 About three months after a TRAM flap with no nipple reconstruction, showing the new breast. A scar in the lower abdomen (the donor site) is also shown.

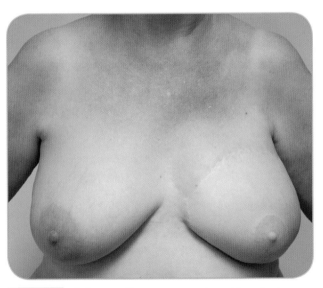

Figure 7.7 A left TRAM flap reconstruction with a nipple reconstruction and a reduction of the right side for balance.

Nipple reconstruction is usually done in one of two ways: your surgeon can use the skin of your reconstruction, raising it and bringing it together to look like a nipple; or "nipple sharing" by transferring part of your nipple from the other side (Figure 7.8). The areola is reconstructed by using a skin graft, usually from the crease of your groin, or is simply tattooed. Neither method will give you a functioning, sensitive nipple; reconstruction is strictly cosmetic.

Table 7.1 Comparison between different types of flap reconstructions

FLAP	LATISSIMUS DORSI	TRAM (PEDICLE)	TRAM (FREE)	DIEP	GLUTEAL
Type of Flap	Pedicle	Pedicle	Free	Free	Free
Donor Site	Upper back	Abdomen	Abdomen	Abdomen	Buttock
Muscle Removed	Yes	Yes	Yes	No	Yes
Suitable with Previous Abdominal Surgery	Definite	Possible	Possible	Possible	Definite
Microsurgery Needed	No	No	Yes	Yes	Yes
Procedure Time (hrs)	2–4	6–8	6–8	6–8	8–12
Days in Hospital	4	7	7	7	7
Smaller Breasted	Yes	Yes	Yes	Yes	Yes
Larger Breasted	Yes, with implant	Yes	Yes	Yes	Yes
Chance of Flap Breakdown or "Necrosis"	Not common	Often minor wound healing problems and partial flap loss	< 5% total flap loss	< 5% total flap loss	< 8% total flap loss
Chance of Abdominal Hernia	No	Yes (<5%)	Yes (<2%)	Yes (<1%)	No
Sensation	No nipple	No nipple	No nipple	No nipple	No nipple

Reconstruction of Your Other Breast

Sometimes your plastic surgeon will talk to you about the other breast. Inevitably, your other breast will not be the same as your reconstructed breast in terms of size and position. Surgery to the other breast can improve symmetry.

This may be a "lift," or mastopexy or a reduction known as a reduction mammoplasty (Figure 7.7), or even an implant to enlarge the other side (Figure 7.5). Removal of the other breast (prophylactic mastectomy) is rarely considered, though we may discuss this difficult choice if you have an exceptionally strong family history of breast cancer and you feel it's easier to have just one anesthetic, remove the burden of constant mammography on that side, and to ensure a symmetrical reconstruction. However, don't rush this decision—it takes a lot of thought and discussion. Always make sure that your plastic surgeon sends any normal tissue from the reduced side for examination by the pathologist.

Recovery after a Reconstruction

You are likely to feel tired and sore for a week or two after implant reconstruction, and for up to three to six weeks after flap procedures. Most of your discomfort can be controlled by painkillers prescribed by your doctor. You'll also have stitches (sutures) in place after your surgery. They'll probably be the kind that dissolve on their own, so you won't need to have them removed.

Depending on the type of surgery, you should be able to leave hospital in one to ten days. Surgical drains are used to remove fluid from the site of your operation. Usually, these drains are removed while you're in the hospital, but you may be discharged with a drain still in place.

Complications and Risks of a Reconstruction

Breast reconstruction carries the possibility of complications. Most commonly, expanders will feel tight until the surrounding tissue stretches. Further, breast implants aren't lifelong devices, and you may eventually need surgery to replace or remove the implant. Also, with breast implants, you could experience complications such as infection or rotation (where the implant moves into the wrong position).

There is a slightly higher risk of infection around the implant with chemotherapy, which may be required in the event that some areas of invasive cancer were found in amongst your DCIS or in the axillary lymph nodes. If your chest wall requires radiation this may increase the risk of **capsulitis**, or capsular contracture. Capsulitis is when scar tissue forms and compresses the implant into a hard and unnatural shape. The odds of this occurring increase in the twelve to twenty-four months after you have had radiation therapy to the chest wall and implant. These complications may require additional surgery and your implant may need to be removed.

Tissue reconstruction is a major procedure. It prolongs your time in surgery and can extend your recovery time by several weeks. Flaps cause pain both at the "donor" site and in the chest area. Removal of muscles from the donor site will cause pain and weakness, or rarely, a hernia.

In addition, poor wound healing, a hernia in your abdominal scar, a collection of fluid (**seroma**) or infection can occur. The worst complication, which is rare, is when the flap doesn't take due to tissue death (a bit like gangrene) from insufficient blood supply. Complications are more common if you are overweight, have diabetes, or are a smoker. As mentioned above, this can occur to a preserved nipple as well if you have a nipple-sparing mastectomy. The nipple may lose its blood supply and parts or all of it may die off.

Should I Have Breast Reconstruction?

Some women find a mastectomy without reconstruction a constant reminder of their DCIS. There is some evidence from the U.K. and the U.S. that you may feel more positive about yourself if you have a reconstruction after a mastectomy. Nevertheless, many women are quite comfortable not having a reconstruction and feel relieved that their DCIS has been removed and the breast is gone. A few days' or even a few weeks' delay in getting treatments that generally take place after surgery will not change your prognosis at all.

Your general health, previous abdominal treatments (which can affect the donor area for a flap reconstruction), your breast size and your own wishes are taken into account to work out which type of reconstruction will give you the best result. The plastic surgeon will give you information on the anesthesia, the location of the operation, and what kind of follow-up procedures may be necessary.

Some women prefer to think about an immediate reconstruction whereas others really just want to have a mastectomy and think about a reconstruction a year or two or even much later. There is no correct answer. Go with not only what is available to you but also with what you feel comfortable doing at this stage. You can always reconsider a reconstruction at a later time.

It's important to understand what you can expect from a breast reconstruction before you make your decision. A reconstruction will not give you a new, normally functioning breast. The difference between your reconstructed and your natural breast will be minimal when you're dressed but usually obvious when you're undressed. Having a reconstruction will provide a contour or shape so that you'll be able to wear most of your usual clothes and swimwear. If you preserve or reconstruct your nipple, the appearance may look more like the other side.

In summary, don't be rushed by your surgeon about this very important decision. It's far better to delay your surgery a week or two and get the right advice than it is to try to conform to your surgeon's operating schedule.

CONTROL POINT #7 – IF I HAVE A MASTECTOMY, WHAT ARE MY OPTIONS FOR BREAST RECONSTRUCTION?

WARNING

There is a chance of nipple involvement from your DCIS if it is large or close to the nipple on your mammogram.

TIP

Don't feel rushed by your surgeon's operating schedule; take the time to work out the best option for you right now. This could include never having a reconstruction, having it done in a few years (delayed reconstruction), or having it done at the same time as your mastectomy (immediate reconstruction).

REMEMBER

Having a breast reconstruction is a very personal decision and you should not be pressured one way or another by your partner, friends, or doctors.

Kerry's Story

My journey with DCIS began around the time my daughter turned one. I found a small, hard lump like a pea, but it didn't show up on a mammogram, which was unusual for DCIS.

After two lumpectomies, a mastectomy was discussed. I was 38 and considering the removal of a breast when I felt fit and healthy except for one little, hard lump. I thought I must be crazy. I was more concerned about being around for the long haul, given the young ages of my children, than I was about keeping my breast; and so in the end, after several weeks of deliberation, I decided to have a mastectomy. The main reason for this decision was my long-term management. How do you monitor a person for a recurrence if their initial DCIS wasn't visible on a mammogram?

My memories of that time are associated with fear, confusion, and the oppressive, looming need to make a decision. The fear was born out of being a young mother wanting so desperately to see my two children grow up. The confusion was related to the fact that while this was a very early stage cancer, or "precancerous condition" as one young intern labeled it, a mastectomy was being contemplated. The need for me as a person and us as a family to make the right decision, one that we could live every day of our lives with, was an incredible burden, but ultimately, I'm glad to have had the choice.

Once I had made the decision and had the surgery, a great weight lifted from me. Six weeks after my mastectomy, my son started school. This month he graduated from high school. I have never regretted my decision but making it was one of the most difficult things in my life.

WHAT IS PAGET'S DISEASE OF THE NIPPLE?

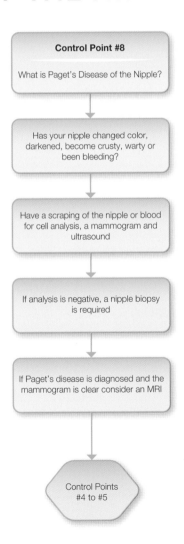

Control Point #8

What is Paget's Disease of the Nipple?

Has your nipple changed color, darkened, become crusty, warty or been bleeding?

Have a scraping of the nipple or blood for cell analysis, a mammogram and ultrasound

If analysis is negative, a nipple biopsy is required

If Paget's disease is diagnosed and the mammogram is clear consider an MRI

Control Points #4 to #5

What Is Paget's Disease of the Nipple?

Paget's disease of the nipple is an uncommon nipple rash where DCIS spreads in or around the nipple (Figure 8.1). It was the French surgeon Valpeau who first described several patients with increasing redness of the nipple (Velpeau 1856). Sir James Paget, from England, however, noted a link between changes in the appearance of the nipple and underlying breast cancer (Paget 1874). Paget wrote the following:

> I believe it has not yet been published that certain chronic affections of the skin of the nipple and areola are very often succeeded by the formation of scirrhous cancer in the mammary gland. I have seen about fifteen cases in which this has happened, and the events were in all of them so similar that one description may suffice.
>
> The patients were all women, various in age from forty to sixty or more years, having in common nothing remarkable but their disease. In all of them the disease began as an eruption on the nipple and areola. In the majority it had the appearance of a florid, intensely red, raw surface, very finely granular, as if nearly the whole thickness of the epidermis were removed; like the surface of very acute diffuse eczema . . . .
>
> From such a surface, on the whole or greater part of the nipple and areola, there was always copious, clear, yellowish, viscid exudation. The sensations were commonly tingling, itching, and burning, but the malady was never attended by disturbance of the general health. I have not seen this form of eruption extend beyond the areola, and only once have seen it pass into a deeper ulceration of the skin after the manner of a rodent ulcer.

He noted that:

> The formation of cancer has not in any case taken place first in the diseased part of the skin. It has always been in the substance of the mammary gland, beneath or not far from the diseased skin, and always with a clear interval of apparently healthy tissue.

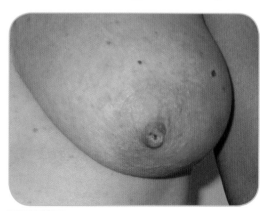

Figure 8.1 Paget's disease of the nipple.

More than 95% of people with Paget's disease of the nipple also have underlying DCIS or an actual breast cancer somewhere in the breast (Figure 8.2, right). Cases where there is no underlying invasive cancer do occur, so trying to sort out whether the nipple rash is just the tip of the iceberg or the whole iceberg is a critical first step (Figure 8.2, left and middle). We don't really know how Paget's disease occurs. I suspect that most cases start off as high-grade DCIS inside the breast ducts and then spread up towards the nipple and then outside it onto the areola. Some patients I have seen just have pure DCIS in the nipple or just below the nipple. In many ways, however, it is academic, as we still need to search very hard inside your breast with imaging tests (mammography, ultrasound, and MRI) to make sure of the true extent of the DCIS and to look for any hidden invasive cancer.

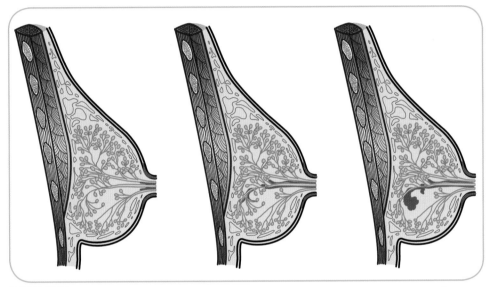

Figure 8.2 Paget's disease of the nipple—(left) nipple only; (center) nipple and major ducts involved with DCIS; (right) nipple, DCIS and invasive cancer.

The European Institute of Oncology in Milan, Italy, studied 114 patients who underwent surgery after presenting with Paget's disease of the nipple from 1996 to 2003 (Caliskan et al. 2008). The average age was 54 years with a range between 27 to 88 years. Of the 114 patients, the following associated tumors were found in the breast:

- None, Paget's disease only: 7 patients (6%)
- DCIS only: 39 patients (34%)
- invasive cancer: 68 patients (60%).

How Common Is Paget's Disease of the Nipple?

Paget's disease of the nipple probably accounts for less than 1% of all breast cancers. Most patients diagnosed with Paget's disease of the nipple are over the age of 50, but, as in the Italian study, rare cases have been diagnosed in patients in their 20s. I have treated Paget's disease in an elderly man as well.

From 1988 to 2002, 1,704 female patients with Paget's disease were recorded in the U.S. SEER cancer registry, of which 51% had an underlying invasive cancer; 36% had an underlying DCIS; and 13% had Paget's disease alone in the nipple without an underlying breast abnormality. The U.S. registry data are very similar to the Italian data above. The average age at diagnosis was higher in the U.S. at 62 years. Its incidence was only 6 cases per 1,000,000 women in 2002 (Chen et al 2006).

What Are the Symptoms of Paget's Disease of the Nipple?

The main sign of Paget's disease of the nipple is a change in the nipple and/or areola, including the following:

- The nipple area might appear velvety red. This is usually the first sign of Paget's disease. I examine the nipple with the help of an examination light and look for differences in color between the two nipples. The color changes are often very subtle and hard to see.

- The nipple area might become harder, scaly or crusty—it may look like dermatitis or eczema. The changes are usually on one side only. If the rash involves both nipples it is probably dermatitis or psoriasis. With time, the changes can spread onto the areola.

- There may be an ulcer or a crack in the skin (fissure) and a clear or bloody discharge from the nipple with a stain on the bra or nightwear.

- The nipple might flatten out or invert inwards. Nipple inversion needs to be new to be of concern. If you have had lifelong nipple inversion, this is not of concern.

- The area might feel itchy, tingly, more sensitive or sore and there may be a lump in the same breast or armpit.

Upon clinical examination, I tend to see a spectrum of changes ranging from redness and slight scaling, which then progresses to crusting, to a superficial skin erosion and then a deeper ulcer. Yellowish fluid can fill the ulcer or a clear or bloody discharge may be evident. Sometimes there is a cancerous lump right behind the nipple and thickening and a leathery feel of the areola from the cancer invading this area. These days, I hardly ever see the Paget's disease extend from the nipple to involve all of the areola or even skin of the breast. In perhaps up to six of ten patients with Paget's disease of the nipple, a lump can be felt in the breast during physical examination (Günhan-Bilgen & Oktay 2006).

Is Paget's Disease of the Nipple Visible on Breast X-rays ?

When Paget's disease is highly suspected, I normally start off by arranging a mammogram and an ultrasound of both breasts. In the series from the European Institute of Oncology, 86% of women with underlying invasive cancer had a change in their mammogram compared to 62% who only had Paget's disease with DCIS.

In a well-conducted study from Turkey, correlation between the clinical presentation and the final pathology and imaging findings was undertaken (Günhan-Bilgen & Oktay 2006). Seventeen women presented with typical nipple changes of Paget's disease and six of the seventeen (35%) were also found to have a breast lump. Two of the seventeen women (12%) had a discharge of blood coming from their nipple.

After a mammogram and ultrasound, findings were as follows:

- normal: 7 (41%)
- abnormal: 10 (59%)
  - microcalcifications only: 3 (18%)
  - mass (lump) with or without calcification: 7 (41%).

The results of the initial mammogram and ultrasound will determine what tests you need next. If the mammogram and ultrasound are normal, a breast MRI may be helpful but at the same time, a biopsy of the nipple skin can be arranged. Figure 1.12 (on page 24) is an MRI of patient who presented with Paget's disease of the nipple with an abnormal mammogram but a large area of underlying DCIS was visible on her MRI.

What Biopsy Tests Do I Need?

If your mammogram and ultrasound do not show any changes, then your surgeon will need to think of how to sample the nipple or its underlying ducts. Different approaches are possible but include:

- Scrape cytology: Here we scrape off some cells from the nipple erosion or ulcer and wipe them on a glass pathology slide. It's a bit like a Pap test. The pathologist then looks at the cells under the microscope.

- Nipple discharge cytology: If you have blood coming out of one of your ducts, this can be wiped onto a glass pathology slide and examined under the microscope

- Wedge biopsy of the nipple: This can be done using a local anesthetic but is more commonly done under general anesthetic where a small sliver of the nipple, underlying ducts, and even a small piece of the areola and underlying breast tissue is removed for a more thorough examination. It is done in such a way that the nipple will still look quite normal if it turns out that the nipple changes are benign.

- If you only have a bloody nipple discharge and your mammogram is clear, a special procedure can be done called a **ductogram**; dye is injected into the duct where the blood is coming from and a mammogram is then taken to see if there are any abnormalities inside the duct. These are sometimes called "filling defects." If there is a filling defect, sometimes the only way to diagnose the abnormality is for a surgeon to perform a **microdochectomy**. This involves two steps. First, immediately before your surgery, the involved duct is found by the radiologist and contrast dye visible on a mammogram is injected into the discharging duct (a ductogram) to find the abnormal filling defects again. Second, you will be taken to the operating room to have the affected duct identified and excised, along with the breast tissue or lobule connected to it. If DCIS is found, you may then need further surgery to the area with or without removal of the nipple region.

If your mammogram is abnormal with microcalcifications only, then the first step is usually a stereotactic-guided core biopsy as previously discussed in "Control Point #1 – What on Earth Is DCIS?" In the series of seventeen patients mentioned above, all seven patients with microcalcification had pure DCIS without any hidden invasive cancer (Günhan-Bilgen & Oktay 2006). If the calcification is close to the nipple, there may be no need to diagnose the nipple area as it will need to be removed whether you have conservative surgery or a mastectomy. If the calcium is more than 2–3 cm from the nipple, then it makes more sense to diagnose the calcium spots with a core biopsy and the nipple change with a scraping test or a wedge biopsy.

If your mammogram and ultrasound showed a lump (mass), then a core biopsy of the lump is vital to exclude an invasive cancer as this will affect what needs to be done to your nodes. Once again, if the lump is away from the nipple and conservation of the breast is planned, it makes sense to find out what the change in the nipple actually is. If it is Paget's disease, then it should also be removed. In Günhan-Bilgen's study, most women (85%) who presented with Paget's disease of the nipple who were found to have a mass on their mammogram or ultrasound ended up having invasive cancer. So, the best situation to be in is where there is no lump to feel and the mammogram shows only calcification.

When a wedge excision of the nipple is taken, a pathologist examines the tissue under a microscope to see if Paget cells are present (Figure 8.3, left). Other cells that may be present are skin lining cells called **keratin** produced by cells called keratinocytes and inflammatory cells called lymphocytes. Pathologists use special stains called immunohistochemistry to help them differentiate Paget's disease from benign disease and types of skin cancer. Most DCIS associated with Paget's disease is high grade and usually estrogen receptor negative. The Paget cells tend to be HER2 positive (Figure 8.3, right), and it has been found that a stain called CK7 tends to be positive and CK20 tends to be negative. The Paget cells also tend to be S100 negative. S100 is a protein stain which is present if it were a type of skin cancer called melanoma of the nipple region.

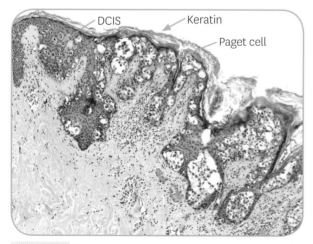
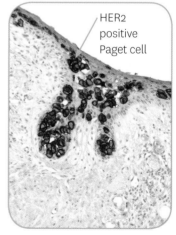

Figure 8.3 Right: Pathology section of the nipple showing keratin (which causes crusting of the nipple) and the large Paget cell; left: Paget's cells are HER2 positive—the brown cells, in the nipple.

How Is Paget's Disease of the Nipple Treated?

Treatment depends on whether there is an underlying DCIS only or an associated invasive cancer and how much of the breast is affected.

Conservative Surgery Alone

Surgery is the most common treatment for Paget's disease of the nipple. Removing the nipple and areola using a procedure called a **central wedge excision** (also known as cone excision) has been used. This procedure removes the nipple, areola, and underlying breast tissue. One study from the U.K. showed that, without radiotherapy, DCIS or invasive cancer came back after this procedure in four of ten patients (40%) (Dixon et al. 1991). Three of the four had invasive cancer, and two of the three subsequently died of breast cancer. I would only recommend this approach if you or your relative are quite old or frail and cannot tolerate a mastectomy or a three- to five-week course of radiation. For example, if you are in your late 80s or in your 90s this could be a good option.

Radiation Alone

Radiation treatment alone for patients with Paget's disease without a palpable mass or abnormal mammogram has been reported; however, widespread experience with such conservative treatment remains limited. One of the largest studies with the longest follow-up time is from France (Forquet et al. 1987). Between 1960 and 1984, twenty selected patients with Paget's disease of the breast confined to the nipple were treated conservatively with radiotherapy alone (seventeen patients) or limited surgery and radiotherapy (three patients). After an average follow-up time of seven and a half years, three of the twenty patients (15%) had recurrence in the breast and were treated with a mastectomy. All recurrences were located in the nipple or areola, and all were Paget's disease without associated DCIS or invasive carcinoma. No patients died of breast disease. I would not normally recommend this sort of approach unless you or your relative cannot tolerate a local or general anesthetic for a very good reason.

Conservative Surgery and Radiation

If your disease is confined to the nipple and the surrounding area, you may undergo breast-conserving surgery, which involves removal of the nipple and areola followed by a three- to six-week course of radiation (see "Control Point #16 – Do I Need Radiation Therapy?"). In a U.S. study of Paget's disease presenting as a nipple abnormality only, the ten-year risk of a recurrence in the breast was 11% when treated with surgery and radiation; of these, half were pure DCIS and half invasive cancer. The ten-year survival free of disease was 97% (Marshall et al. 2003). Between 1987 and 1998, sixty-one eligible patients were registered in the European Organization for Research and Treatment of Cancer Study (EORTC) 10873. Nearly all patients (97%) presented without an associated palpable mass. At histologic examination, the majority (93%) of patients had an underlying area of DCIS in the breast; and in the remaining 7%, only Paget's disease was found.

Treatment was complete excision of the nipple-areolar complex, including the underlying breast tissue with tumor-free margins, followed by five weeks of radiation to the whole breast. At a median follow-up of just over six years, four of the sixty-one patients (6.6%) developed a recurrence in the treated breast (one patient with DCIS and three patients with invasive disease). The overall survival rate was over 98% (Bijker et al. 2001). In other words, following wide local excision and radiation therapy, the chance of another recurrence is, at most, one in ten.

Total Mastectomy with or without Reconstruction

A total mastectomy may be recommended when there is extensive DCIS (generally more than 4 to 5 cm), if there are multiple areas of DCIS or invasive cancer in the breast, or if you just feel more comfortable having a mastectomy. A reconstruction may be considered either immediately or delayed until a year or more after your mastectomy (see "Control Point #7– If I Have a Mastectomy, What Are My Options for Breast Reconstruction?") I nearly always recommend a sentinel node biopsy in this setting. In the Italian study noted above, of the twenty-one patients who had a mastectomy and had Paget's disease with only underlying DCIS, only one patient developed a recurrence on the skin of the chest wall and one developed recurrence in a lymph node in the armpit. The long-term survival rate, free of breast cancer, was over 95% (Caliskan et al. 2008). If it turns out that you had an invasive cancer, then your treatment will be more complicated as decisions need to be made about what to do with the remainder of the lymph nodes in your armpit as well as decisions about chemotherapy and hormonal treatment. Please see my first book called *Breast Cancer: Taking Control*.

Skin-Sparing Mastectomy

This procedure was explained in "Control Point #4 – What Will I Do about My Breast?" The technique essentially leaves more skin and uses smaller scars, allowing an implant or muscle flap to be inserted at the first operation. As Paget's disease involves the nipple, a nipple-sparing mastectomy is contraindicated.

All other things being equal, my favored approach is to try and remove the nipple and areola with clear margins and then add a course of radiation therapy.

Should I Have a Sentinel Node Biopsy?

Patients with Paget's disease and a known invasive cancer should be offered a sentinel node biopsy to evaluate their nodal status. If the imaging is clear, with disease only in the nipple, and breast conservation is to be performed, a sentinel node biopsy could be done at a later date if invasive disease was identified. Some clinicians may recommend a sentinel node biopsy at the outset for all patients with Paget's disease given that at least six out of ten patients have an underlying invasive cancer. If a mastectomy is to be performed, a sentinel node biopsy should be done at the time of surgery due to the possibility that invasive cancer may be identified in the mastectomy specimen, making it virtually impossible to do a sentinel node biopsy later as there is no breast tissue to inject the radioactive dye into. "See Control Point #5 – What Will I Do about My Armpit?"

CONTROL POINT #8 – WHAT IS PAGET'S DISEASE OF THE NIPPLE?

 Paget's disease is often a sign of an underlying DCIS or invasive cancer in your breast.

 If your mammogram and ultrasound are clear, it is a good idea to have a breast MRI.

 The survival rates for a mastectomy or removal of the nipple and areola followed by radiation are the same.

Aly's Story

Four years ago, aged 66, I went to my GP for a checkup. She noticed a small flake of skin on my left nipple and said it was Paget's disease, which she had only seen once before. I checked my breasts for lumps regularly and had seen the dry skin but thought nothing of it. Occasionally, skin had fallen off and there had been a drop of blood. I had a mammogram and ultrasound and saw a dermatologist who took a biopsy.

Because of the Christmas holiday period, I didn't get the results of the biopsy for three weeks, which was an anxious time. I was referred to a surgeon who removed the nipple and underlying tissue and DCIS. I also had a sentinel node biopsy.

After the surgery, I was surprised at how mild the pain was and that only three lymph nodes were removed, which made it less intrusive. The nursing care I received was excellent. There were more tests, and I saw a radiation oncologist regarding radiotherapy. I was to have six weeks' treatment and had three dots tattooed on my chest to align the equipment. The radiotherapy treatments were very quick once everything was aligned, and, on most days, I was in and out in fifteen minutes.

I felt quite tired for a few months but am now so much better that I rarely think of it; and so little tissue was removed that I don't notice it. I see both my surgeon and oncologist every year and, so far, after four years everything is clear. I was advised that, after a period of one year, my GP could check me once a year with a breast exam and breast X-rays.

WHAT SHOULD I DO BEFORE I GO TO THE HOSPITAL?

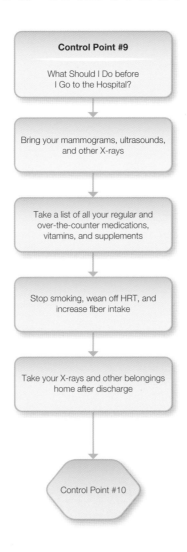

Control Point #9

What Should I Do before
I Go to the Hospital?

↓

Bring your mammograms, ultrasounds,
and other X-rays

↓

Take a list of all your regular and
over-the-counter medications,
vitamins, and supplements

↓

Stop smoking, wean off HRT, and
increase fiber intake

↓

Take your X-rays and other belongings
home after discharge

↓

Control Point #10

9

Tips: Before Going to the Hospital

Going to the hospital, particularly for the first time, can be frightening and overwhelming. This chapter will give you some ideas to make your hospital stay a little easier. Your doctor or nurse will also give you specific information about the hospital you'll be going to.

- Stop smoking as soon as possible. Speak to your doctor about nicotine gum or patches to combat cravings and urges to smoke.

- Stop taking aspirin, contraceptive pills, hormone (replacement) therapy, and green tea as these can influence clotting. Talk to your team to see what they advise.

- If you are a diabetic, be diligent about monitoring your sugar levels before going to the hospital.

- Take a list of all your regular medications and over-the-counter preparations.

- Eat well before you go to the hospital; take fiber because you can get constipated lying around in a hospital bed.

- Take your identification and health cards (e.g., Medicare or insurance card) and the name, address, and contact numbers of your family doctor and specialist.

- Bring details of past illnesses (dates and diagnoses) and a list of allergies.

- Bring your mammograms, ultrasounds, and other X-rays, but don't forget to take them home with you. Write your phone number on the X-ray packet just in case it is misplaced.

- Get details on the costs of treatment, including the specialist, anesthetist, pathologist, and hospital fees.

- Find out what time to arrive, where to go, and how long you need to fast beforehand.

- Take glasses or contact lenses and eye drops, if needed.

- Bring your cell phone, address book, portable music player, iPad or tablet, and portable computer (and DVDs if you'll have a long stay); and don't forget your power cords, chargers, and a power strip (if needed).

- Bring cash for phone calls, the coffee shop, etc., but leave jewelry at home.

- Pack toiletries, including toothbrush, soap, shampoo, face wipes, and aluminum-free deodorant. Aluminum is thought to make skin reaction from radiation therapy worse.

- Pack makeup and a hair dryer, if desired.

- Pack slippers, a comfy robe, and pajamas if you're staying for more than one day. Button-up pajamas are slightly more practical than nightgowns.

- Pack reading material, such as books and magazines.

- Take your pillow, quilt cover, or perhaps a familiar cushion or a throw rug for the visitor's chair.

- Take photos of family or loved ones.

- Take a couple of bottles of your favorite water because the hospital air conditioning can dry out your throat.

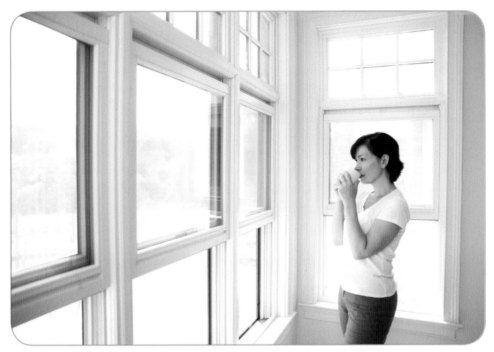

Going to the hospital can be frightening and overwhelming.

Tips: Upon Arrival at the Hospital

When you arrive at the hospital for the first time, you will need to check in at the admissions office, which is usually near the main entrance.

Find out about:

- access you might have to television, radio, newspapers, or the Internet

- access you might have to storage of any valuables

- the hospital's visitor policy and visiting times, and where your visitors can park

- when you can expect to be discharged, from where (as some hospitals have a discharge lounge), and at what time.

Once in your hospital room, work out how to use the call system between you and the nurse, as well as telephones and the bed controls.

It's not unusual to feel weak or tired while in the hospital, so use the call button when you need help. Be careful not to trip over wires or tubes when you get in or out of bed. It's best to keep your things within easy reach. Make sure you hold onto support bars when getting in or out of the bath or shower, and use the handrails on stairways and in hallways. Most doctors and hospitals now encourage early mobilization to get your feet and legs moving to prevent blood clots.

Tips for the Elderly

Hospital stays can be quite disorienting, particularly for the elderly when removed from their usual environment. If you are a family member reading this, please be aware that older people (particularly those over 75–80 years) can drift from being relatively independent to dependent in a surprisingly short period of time. You can help by bringing familiar things to the hospital such as family photos or a favorite pillow or gown. A strange hospital ward can be a very frightening place for the elderly, and you may need to stay overnight with them. Find out how this can be done if required.

CONTROL POINT #9 – WHAT SHOULD I DO BEFORE I GO TO THE HOSPITAL?

 Stop smoking as soon as possible. Eat well before you go into the hospital; take fiber, because you can get constipated lying around in a hospital bed

 Take a list of all your regular medications and over-the-counter preparations.

 Bring your mammograms, ultrasounds, and other X-rays, and don't forget to take them home with you.

CONTROL POINT #10

HOW DO I COPE WITH WAITING FOR MY RESULTS?

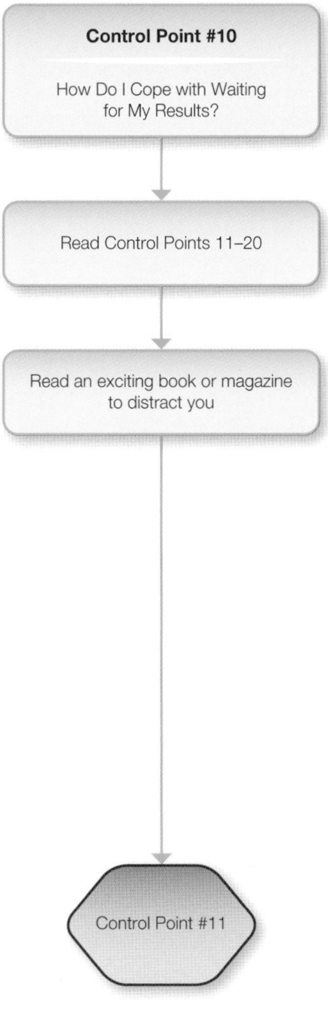

10

Tips While Waiting for Your Results

The week after your surgery will be one of those really bad weeks. I mentioned above that waiting to see the doctor for the first time is a horrible week. Well, this week, waiting around for the results, is even worse. You may be in a state of shock. You may have been rushed into surgery without enough time to get your thoughts and your information together. You may still be coming to terms with what DCIS really means and whether or not there may be an underlying cancer.

Your results will take a while to come through. If you're up to it, start getting your thoughts together before you leave the hospital, and start reading Part 3, the green section, of this book if you have not already done so. Take some control at this point by getting ready for your next doctor's appointment.

A good doctor will talk to you like a real human being and try to give you as much time as possible. That's the good news. The flip side is that they're doing that with all their other patients too, so they'll battle to run their appointments on time. This can be frustrating. Doctors who treat breast cancer usually do not run on time, as it's often unpredictable and difficult to know if a patient will take thirty to sixty minutes or five minutes. In addition, they may have one or two "urgent" cases squeezed onto their list, which makes the waiting times worse.

Like you, other patients will be getting their results on the same day that you are, and most people will have lots of questions. Just as with the doctor, the receptionist often can't predict how long things will take.

Waiting to get your results after your surgery is not only scary, but also very frustrating, and you may feel you are waiting to receive your "sentence." You may experience periods of depression, anger, and hurt as you worry over questions like: Will it be good news or not so good? Will it be more than just DCIS?

Here are some hints to help you cope:

- Talk to your family, friends, and children about your surgery and your feelings.
- Do not be afraid to show your husband or partner your scar, even if you've had a mastectomy. This is a really important but often difficult step for emotional healing.
- Get ready for your postoperative doctor's visit. Have your questions ready and, more importantly, written down. I have some key questions you can ask at the back of this book. Make sure you take that checklist when you see your doctor.

- Reread the first few chapters of this book, which define what DCIS really is.

- Do not be afraid to ask your surgeon directly about his or her preferred method if you receive conflicting advice from different nurses or junior doctors on the ward about how to manage your scar.

- Keep reading your favorite novel or book, or get back on your computer and keep in touch with the outside world. When you go to your doctor's office, take a book or magazine to read, or some craftwork if you are that way inclined, or your iPad to keep you occupied while you wait.

- If you're a person who likes researching your own condition, exercise caution regarding how much information you seek out online. There's a wealth of information out there, but not all of it is good or even right. Some of it will have the potential to scare you or lead you down the wrong path.

- Start walking and try to build up to half an hour a day, three or four times a week.

- Start on a healthy diet, but don't be afraid to have the odd bit of chocolate or treat as a reward, maybe at the end of the week.

- When you have reasonable shoulder movement (and if you have power steering), take yourself for a short drive if you have had only a sentinel node biopsy to your armpit or no treatment to your armpit and are not taking any strong painkillers.

- If you're not taking pain medication, small amounts (one or, at most, two glasses a day) of alcohol are okay.

Tips: Preparing for Your Postoperative Visit to Your Surgeon

Here is a checklist you can take with you to your appointment to help remind you of everything you should ask your doctor.

- Is there any sign of redness or pain around the scar to suggest infection? If there is, consider taking antibiotics for a week.

- Be sure you ask the surgeon for a copy of the pathology report. Ask your surgeon to highlight the following important findings:

  - the size of the DCIS in millimeters or inches

  - the type of DCIS (e.g., solid, cribriform, etc.) (see Figures 1.2–1.5 on page 20)

  - whether the DCIS is one area or multiple areas

  - the margin of normal tissue around the DCIS

  - the **nuclear grade** of the DCIS

  - the presence of necrosis within the DCIS

  - what the calcification on your mammogram was, that is, was it calcified necrosis as part of the DCIS or was it something else (like a benign change)

 – any other change around your DCIS such as hyperplasia or atypia which may indicate an "overactive" or "busy" breast

- Ask about test results that were not available straightaway since some may take an extra few days to come back. These tests are fairly critical for making decisions about **adjuvant**, or additional, therapy over and above the surgery.

The tests you should ask about are:

- the estrogen receptor test, which determines if your DCIS is sensitive to antiestrogen therapies

- the final immunohistochemistry test on your sentinel node biopsy, if this was done

- most importantly, was the pathologist able to see any sign of "microinvasion", or an invasive cancer, in or around the area of DCIS.

Waiting to see your doctor after your surgery for your DCIS is a very anxious time, as you will naturally be worried about the final pathology results; whether or not you will need more surgery; and what other treatments, specifically radiation therapy, chemotherapy, or hormonal treatment, you will need.

There is a lot to discuss at your first postoperative visit. It's best to bring somebody along with you, and even a person who can take some notes. Control Points #11 to #19 discuss the key decisions and steps that you and your doctor will need to think about after your surgery to work out the best treatment— not for some theoretical person in a textbook, but for you and your own individual circumstances.

CONTROL POINT #10 – HOW DO I COPE WITH WAITING FOR MY RESULTS?

WARNING

If you're a person who likes researching your own condition, exercise caution regarding how much information you seek out online. There's a wealth of information out there, but not all of it is good or even right. Some of it will have the potential to scare you or lead you down the wrong path.

TIP

Keep reading your favorite novel or book, or get back on your computer and keep in touch with the outside world. When you go to your doctor's office, take a book or magazine to read, or some craftwork if you are that way inclined, to keep you occupied while you wait.

REMEMBER

Talk to your family, friends, and children about your surgery and your feelings.

Kimberley's Story

This was a really difficult time. Waiting for the results was excruciating because there was nothing that I could do but sit and think about the possibility that the news might be the worst.

It seemed to me that I dripped fear from every pore in my body, and I could almost taste it on my breath. Being that afraid worried me too, because I didn't want my body to be enveloped in such negative feelings when I was trying to overcome cancer.

I rang a Cancer Help Line and predictably burst into tears when talking to them. It did help to talk to them, but I was still scared stiff. Then I read some information about dealing with fear. It said that fear was just really strong anxiety and that being afraid didn't actually achieve anything.

That struck a chord with me. I'd learned to listen to fear because it tells us that we are in a dangerous situation and should do something. But here there was no reason to listen to the fear. Everything that could be done was being done and there was nothing I should do. So I gave myself permission to try my best to ignore my fear. Easier said than done.

I thought about what was the best way to distract myself, and for me that has always been to lose myself in a good book. I hadn't read *The Da Vinci Code*, and so I immersed myself in that and it worked for me. Occasionally, the fear would flood in, but I would just acknowledge it and say, "Yep, I'm afraid, but it's okay not to think about that," and try to refocus.

Of course I was still afraid, but I felt better that I wasn't afraid all the time.

PART 3

"MAINTAINING CONTROL"

TAKING CONTROL AFTER
YOUR SURGERY

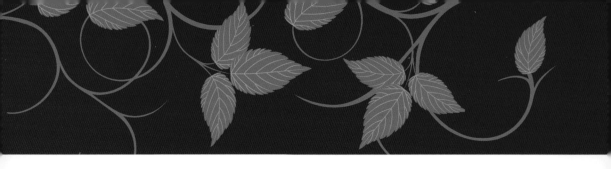

CONTROL POINT #11

HOW DO I ADDRESS ANY POSSIBLE COMPLICATIONS?

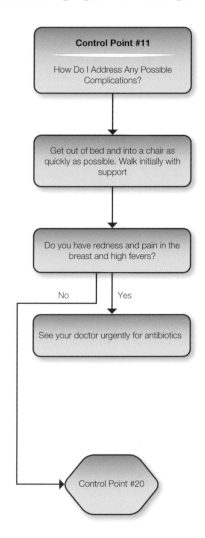

Control Point #11

How Do I Address Any Possible Complications?

↓

Get out of bed and into a chair as quickly as possible. Walk initially with support

↓

Do you have redness and pain in the breast and high fevers?

No   Yes

See your doctor urgently for antibiotics

Control Point #20

11

Common Side Effects after Surgery

Apart from your emotional well-being, coping with your physical side effects and knowing what's normal and what's an unexpected complication of your surgery is really important right now.

The first important step now is to look at the surgical aspects of your breast cancer. The surgeon needs to check your scars and make sure that there's no infection or bruising. If the lymph **glands** have been sampled, there may be a smaller scar in the armpit, or the same scar from your breast may extend into the armpit. Speak to your surgeon before the surgery to find out exactly how many scars or wounds he or she is planning.

If there's a collection of fluid under the armpit or around the scar in your breast called a seroma, then this will need to be drained. It's a fairly minor procedure that can be done straightaway with a needle and syringe by your doctor or nurse. Often the armpit is a little bit numb, and this actually helps lessen the usual stinging you get with an injection.

The wound or wounds will usually be covered by a dressing that can be removed the day after surgery. Underneath the dressing, there may be Steri-Strips. These are small paper tapes that hold the wound in place and usually come off over the next seven to ten days. If they start to peel, don't get too worried. They can be trimmed using a pair of clean scissors.

I am a big fan of using dissolving stitches under the skin. Some surgeons still use staples or sutures outside the skin, but these are really unnecessary and just cause problems later on with more scarring. The good surgeons know how to place the scars along the natural lines of your skin, which are called **Langer's lines**. Doing so aids healing and yields a better cosmetic result.

You won't come to any harm washing your wound, even the day after your surgery. Just make sure that you pat the wound dry using a soft, clean towel. Keeping the area clean, in fact, helps prevent infection and encourages healing.

During surgery a drainage tube, or "drain," may be placed into the scar over your breast or chest area, or into the armpit wound if you had surgery there. This may need to stay in for a few days. Some surgeons use drains that you can drain yourself on a daily basis. If this is the case, keep a record of how much fluid is drained every day. Also, record the color of the fluid, which will slowly change from red, to reddish yellow, to a straw color. We normally remove the drain when less than 25 mL per day drains out over two consecutive days, but please check with your own surgeon. It certainly is a real relief when your drain is out, and you'll feel a lot more comfortable.

On the first day after your surgery, it's good to get up for a walk and sit out of bed. You may need to support your arm when walking or sitting. Practice these exercises:

- deep breathing and coughing to help open up your air passages after anesthetic
- bending and straightening elbows, wrists, and fingers
- bending your ankles and knees to keep your circulation moving
- squeezing your shoulder blades together.

Pain

It is not uncommon to have some pain after breast surgery. Usually, the recommended dosage of acetaminophen/paracetemol (usually branded as Tylenol/Panadol), with or without codeine, is all that you need. If you're experiencing severe pain, then there may be something wrong, such as a collection of normal tissue fluid that causes pressure but is not dangerous. Or, rarely, there may be a collection of pus (an **abscess**), which is more serious and requires urgent drainage and antibiotics.

Bruising

Bruising occurs in about one in ten or twenty patients and may be more common if you're taking a blood-thinning agent. Try not to take any aspirin before your operation. I have now seen two patients who had a lot of bruising, and we discovered that they drank large amounts of green tea. The concern is the high vitamin K content of green tea leaves, which in excessive amounts could potentially interfere with clotting mechanisms and therefore cause bleeding or bruising. Most bruising settles down within a two- to four-week period.

Wound Swelling

It's not uncommon to get some puffiness or firmness around the scar, and occasionally, some fluid may come out of the scar. Again, don't worry too much, but do check with your doctor.

Seroma

Seroma is a collection of fluid that normally occurs under the scar in the armpit region but can also occur under the scar of your breast, or even under a mastectomy scar if your breast was removed. This is normal fluid in your body that has leaked a little bit because of surgery. This can cause a swelling under your armpit (like a golf or tennis ball) that will need to be drained by your surgeon using a needle and syringe or by a radiologist under ultrasound control. A seroma nearly always settles down without further surgery.

Numbness and Loss of Nipple Sensitivity

This is not uncommon and usually decreases, particularly three months after surgery. It can occur around your scar in the breast and in the upper and inner part of your arm if you have had a sentinel node biopsy. You may experience some numbness around the scar on your breast and nipple numbness can occur after surgery, which is close to the nipple or following a nipple-sparing mastectomy. Most women lose nipple sensation and erectile potential of the nipple after a nipple-sparing mastectomy. What you are left with at twelve months is generally what you can expect for the rest of your life.

Uncommon Side Effects after Surgery

Wound Infection

Occasionally, more difficult complications can occur after surgery, such as a wound infection. When this occurs, the wound may become more painful, red, and hot. A diffuse area of infection involving the skin is called **cellulitis**. If the infection gets into the bloodstream, you may become quite ill and run a fever. If you experience these symptoms, it's important to see your doctor immediately and get some antibiotics. While wound infection happens occasionally, it is very uncommon to get a more serious boil or abscess.

Cording

Some women who have a sentinel node biopsy for DCIS have pain, tightness, and a fibrous band that feels like a tight cord running from their armpit to the back of the hand. This is called **cording**. It is thought to be due to hardened lymph vessels. Sometimes it can make it difficult to move the arm. Physiotherapy can help, and sometimes antibiotics are given. I find that regular vitamin E massage of the inner arm can be helpful to ease your symptoms. The pain usually gets better gradually over a few months, but can sometimes come back. A type of cording can also occur along the outside part of the breast. This is called **Mondor's disease**, after the French surgeon who first described the medical syndrome. This is very rare and it is basically a blood clot of one of the superficial veins of the breast. It again presents a slender, often tender and slightly reddened, linear cord just under the skin of the breast. It is sometimes called "sclerosing thrombophlebitis." It can happen as a result of your surgery or, sometimes, it can happen spontaneously. Often the presentation is of the "cording" protruding under the breast but, where it runs through the breast, it pulls it in, creating indentation or puckering and may be confused with what a cancer can look like. Normally if this happens, I recommend some massage with vitamin E or ibuprofen gel. Like most superficial clots, your own body's defenses will get rid of it with time.

Wound Problems

You sometimes find you are left with a fatty lump at the outer edge of the scar under your armpit. This lumpy area usually settles over a period of time. Occasionally, this extra tissue (called a "dog ear") may need to be trimmed at a later date. Wound breakdown is uncommon and means that the scar does not look clean, may be red and swollen, and can come apart, which can delay the healing process from a few days to up to about three weeks. More often than not, it's because the blood supply to a small area of skin has been compromised and the wound doesn't heal properly in that area. The body heals this area by forming a scab, which eventually falls off. This is particularly a problem after a skin-sparing or nipple-sparing mastectomy. Very rarely, this area may need to be removed by a small operation. Very rarely, the whole nipple will have to be removed because of a compromised blood supply. It may be more frequent in people who smoke, and apart from an increased chance of chest problems if you smoke, this is another reason why it's a good idea to quit before your surgery. Once your wound is healed, we advise our patients to massage their scar and surrounding skin with Bio-Oil in a circular motion, twice a day, for a minimum period of three months. This is used to help improve the appearance of your scar.

Call your doctor or breast care nurse immediately if you have:

- a temperature over 38.0 °C or 100.4 °F

- signs of infection such as redness, pain, or swelling

- signs of an extensive bruise (**hematoma**)

- chest pain and shortness of breath, which may indicate a heart attack or a blood clot in the calf traveling to the chest.

The most important thing is to try not to stress too much. Most problems that arise after breast surgery are not emergencies, and they can be managed by you or your family doctor.

CONTROL POINT #11 – HOW DO I ADDRESS ANY POSSIBLE COMPLICATIONS?

WARNING

If you have a temperature over 38.0 °C or 100.4 °F or any signs of infection such as redness, pain, or swelling, see your doctor immediately for antibiotics.

TIP

On the first day after your surgery, it's good to get up for a walk and sit out of bed. You may need to support your arm when walking or sitting.

REMEMBER

The most important thing is to try not to stress too much. Most problems that arise after breast surgery are not emergencies, and they can be managed by you or your family doctor

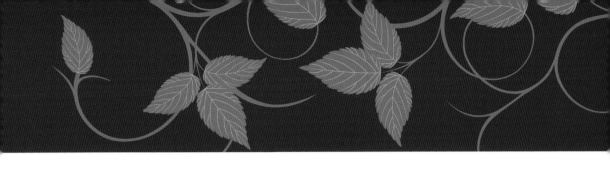

CONTROL POINT #12

DO I NEED MORE SURGERY?

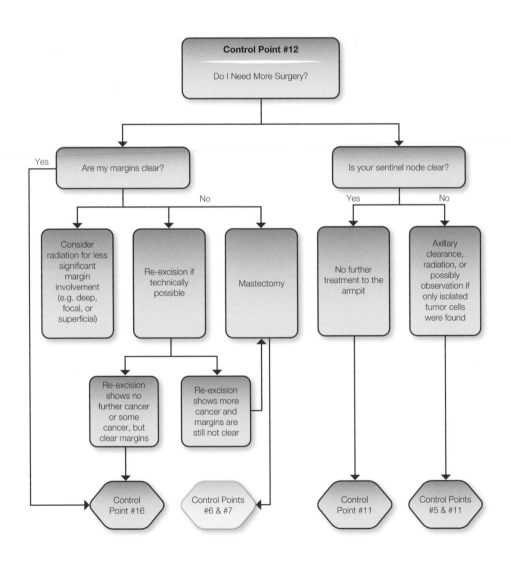

Do I Need More Surgery?

The next important question is: "Do I need any more surgery?" There are two key aspects right now to consider following surgery to your breast and possibly your axilla. It is a particularly stressful time when you need to go back to your doctor's office to be given your results. Make sure you take a support person with you at this very important visit.

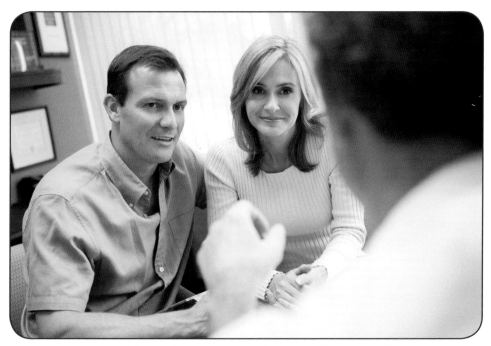

Take a support person with you when you go to see the surgeon for your results.

Are My Margins Clear?

During breast conservation surgery, the surgeon often removes a piece of tissue the size of a golf ball, or even larger. The specimen is then labeled by the surgeon using either sutures or inks to tell the pathologist the orientation of the specimen within the breast. This is important for the pathologist to work out what is going on in the margin, or edge, of the specimen. The margin is the distance between your invasive cancer or any precancer (DCIS) and the edge of the tissue that has been removed. If you have had a lumpectomy, then it is important that you have a clear margin, but there's a lot of debate about what a clear margin actually is. I remember reading an article a long time ago from a famous pathologist who claimed that in order to examine all the margins in a sphere of breast tissue, you need over 3,000 thin sections taken for each patient, which would be an impossible task (Carter 1986). So the margins are just one element of what we look at. Other factors include:

- patient factors: your age and general condition, your motivation to keep your breast, how large your breast is, and whether or not it can tolerate more surgery

- tumor factors: the type of DCIS (e.g., papillary DCIS tends to be more widespread than meets the eye, so it's always best to re-excise)

- treatment factors: which margin is involved, the appearance of the specimen mammogram, and whether or not radiation will be given.

There is a lot of debate about how deep or wide the surgical resection margins need to be after treatment for DCIS. I accept margins as small as 0.5 mm or even less for patients with invasive breast cancer as long as there are no other factors that may result in a higher chance of cancer coming back and the patient is receiving radiation. However, patients with invasive disease are often receiving other treatments such as chemotherapy and hormonal treatment that can make the radiation work better with closer margins.

However, a big problem is that, until very recently, there was little consensus about what constitutes a negative margin (Taghian et al. 2005). There is now increasing evidence that a margin of 2 mm is preferred if you only have DCIS. A very good study from the Memorial Sloan-Kettering Cancer Center, New York, examined all the publications which documented the distance between the surgical cut and the DCIS and the risk of DCIS or cancer coming back in the breast after surgery and radiation. Recurrence rates in the breast were slightly higher if the margin was less than 2 mm (Dunne et al. 2009).

Rates of recurrence in the breast were as follows:

- 1 mm or less: about 10%

- 2 mm: 6%

- 5 mm or more: 4%.

The real point is that wider and wider margins may make the surgeon feel better, but in reality the recurrence rates are no better in the breast and larger margins mean a greater cosmetic deformity.

So if you have DCIS treated by a lumpectomy, also known as a wide local excision, then 2 mm margins appear adequate if radiation is going to be given after your surgery. However, this 2 mm margin cannot be a hard-and-fast rule particularly if:

- your margin, which is close or indeed positive, is the deep margin and the surgeon has taken away the breast tissue in that region down to the pectoral muscle. A mastectomy or re-excision will not help in this setting. Radiation therapy easily gets down that far.

- you had a specimen mammogram, and your specimen was potentially compressed by the so-called "pancake effect" (Graham et al. 2002). In this study, it was found that a 10 mm margin could be reduced to 2.5 mm by the compression, which is used at the time of the specimen mammogram

- your involved margin is superficial, particularly if some skin above the DCIS has already been removed

- your margin, which is less than 2 mm, has normal ducts between the DCIS and the cut surgical edge

- you are elderly and have other conditions which may be more serious than your DCIS

- you are receiving radiation to the whole breast, possibly including an extra dose or **boost**

- the only finding is lobular carcinoma in situ (LCIS) (Ciocca et al. 2008).

I would certainly be more inclined to recommend a re-excision of the area if:

- there is indication of extensive high-grade DCIS

- there are multiple close margins

- the surrounding tissue is not DCIS but still quite abnormal with extensive hyperplasia or atypia

- you are very young or have a strong family history

- a post-excision mammogram shows residual worrying calcifications.

Moving away for the moment from all the "data," if cancer is touching the edge of the surgical cut, this is known as a "positive" or "dirty" margin. In Figures 12.1 and 12.2, I have used a fried egg to clarify what I mean by a clear or "negative" and a close or "positive" margin. The egg yolk represents the DCIS, and the egg white the margin of normal breast tissue around the DCIS. If you have a positive margin or a margin less than 2 mm, then you may need an extra "shave" of tissue removed in the area where the margin was positive. Sometimes a mastectomy may be required but usually the surgeon can go back in and do a re-excision first. A mastectomy can always be done later even after two re-excision procedures if your breast is large enough to allow more tissue to be removed because of a positive margin. I find it frustrating, when I hear of cases having a mastectomy for a positive or close margin, and then the

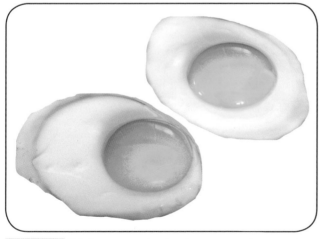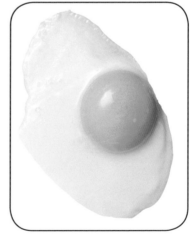

Figure 12.1 This is an example of a clear, or negative, margin on the top right and a close margin on the bottom left. **Figure 12.2** Egg yolk extending to the edge of the white is like a positive margin.

final pathology report of the whole breast shows no disease at all. In some circumstances, when an extra margin cannot be obtained with more surgery or when the margin involvement is minimal or "focal," radiotherapy can also be given.

Do I Need a Post-Excision Mammogram?

This sounds worse than it really is, so don't panic if your doctor wants to repeat the mammogram after your initial surgery. If there is real doubt that areas of calcium may have been left behind, a post-excision mammogram may help decide whether the surgeon should go back and re-excise where your DCIS started. The information that we need to correlate are your:

- initial mammogram
- initial magnification views
- specimen mammogram
- **macroscopic report** (see "Control Point #13 – What Does My Pathology Report Really Mean?")
- final microscopic pathology report.

Once the post-excision mammogram is done, we look for any residual calcium specks by comparing the new mammogram done after your surgery to your initial mammogram. If calcium specks are left behind, we have to make a decision about more surgery. One method of helping this decision is determining if all the calcium seen in your final pathology report is due to DCIS (as shown in Figure 1.3, on page 20), or is it in areas which are not DCIS? So it can be a difficult decision. If your surgeon and oncologist are not sure, they may recommend a re-excision or sometimes even a mastectomy.

In one study from Roswell Park Cancer Institute, sixty-seven patients had a post-excision mammogram and nearly one-quarter were found to have residual microcalcifications. Of the women who had residual calcification and had more surgery, 64% had residual DCIS (Waddell et al. 2000). I also sometimes advise a postoperative breast MRI if I'm not sure, particularly for patients with high-grade DCIS. Figure 1.12 is such an example showing residual invasive cancer of the breast.

Do I Need to Have My Other Breast Taken Off?

The short answer is no in most situations. Patients with DCIS have a slightly increased risk of contra-lateral breast cancer, with an annual rate of approximately six in one thousand per year (Tuttle et al. 2009). With eight years of follow-up data from the National Surgical Adjuvant Breast and Bowel Project (NSABP) B17, Fisher reported that 4.3% of patients who underwent breast conservation for DCIS developed breast cancer in the other side with a risk of eight per thousand per year.

In another study from Fisher, the NSABP (B-24), approximately two-thirds of contralateral breast cancers after conservative surgery and radiation were invasive cancers (Wapnir et al. 2011). This study also found that tamoxifen reduced the risk of opposite breast cancer. I will discuss the role of tamoxifen in reducing contralateral invasive cancer or DCIS in "Control Point #17 – Do I Need Hormonal Treatment?"

Using the SEER database of 18,845 patients with DCIS, Gao et al. (2003) reported that the risk of breast cancer in the other normal breast increased with time (five years, 3.3%; ten years, 6.0%; fifteen years, 8.7%; twenty years, 10.6%), but the annual risk was relatively constant at about five per one thousand per year. This may be higher if you have a family history of breast cancer or if you have been on HRT.

But note, taking the other breast off has not been shown to improve overall survival rates in this setting, and I would restrict a serious discussion about this approach to you if you have a very strong family history. In the updated publication from SEER, there is no doubt that there has been a major increase in the use of prophylactic mastectomy (Tuttle et al. 2009). Among patients who underwent mastectomy to treat DCIS (excluding patients undergoing breast-conserving surgery), the use of a prophylactic mastectomy of the opposite healthy side increased from 6.4% in 1998 to a staggering 18.4% in 2005.

Many factors have probably contributed to the increased removal of the other breast for DCIS. The availability of genetic counseling and testing has increased in recent years. Improvements in breast reconstruction and oncoplastic surgical techniques have also been responsible for this. Also, because obesity has increased in Western societies, obese women with larger breasts may choose to have their normal breast removed to avoid imbalance and asymmetry. The increased use of breast MRI may also have contributed to this nearly tripling of the use of contralateral prophylactic mastectomy.

Is My Sentinel Node Biopsy Clear?

The next decision that needs to be made is whether or not you require more surgery for the lymph glands under your armpit. You may recall from earlier that the sentinel node is thought to be the first draining lymph node that acts as a filter trap for any cancer cells that may have spread from the cancer in your breast, and that the surgeon usually does a quick test on your sentinel node while you're asleep.

Unfortunately, the quick test is only about 50% accurate, and even after a negative quick test, some patients do receive the disappointing news that the final sentinel node test shows some cancer cells. This is called a "positive sentinel node" (Figure 5.5 on page 77). In Hanna's story (see "Control Point #13 – What Does My Pathology Report Really Mean?"), you can see she only had fourteen cells involved in the sentinel node. We made a decision to treat the breast with radiation and cover the glands in level 1 of the axilla (Figure 5.1 on page 73) just with radiation rather than sending her back for more surgery.

In a review of the literature using a meta-analysis technique, van Deurzen et al. (2008) found twenty-nine studies containing 836 patients who had an axillary dissection after they were found to have isolated tumor cells (ITCs) in their sentinel node. The overall positivity rate of the non-sentinel nodes was 12% and two-thirds of these were actual macrometastases, or cancer that was over 2 mm in the lymph node.

In this situation, the surgeon may book you in for an axillary clearance (where the surgeon goes back and takes out some or all of the rest of your lymph glands in your armpit) in the next week or so, or he or she may make a decision not to put you through any more surgery.

The sentinel node testing protocol by the examining pathologist is so thorough that we often detect cancer cells that we didn't even know existed perhaps five or ten years ago. So please don't be too concerned if your sentinel node is involved. It may indeed be the only node involved, or if it only shows a "touch of cancer" (or, to use the medical word, a micrometastasis or isolated tumor cells, ITCs), then the chances of other lymph glands being involved may be very low. Recent **clinical trials** strongly suggest that it is safe not to dissect your axilla if only an ITC or a micrometastasis is found particularly for patients having radiation therapy who are aged over 50 (Giuliano 2010).

If a sentinel node is definitely involved, and particularly if a pathologist can see the cancer cells without the assistance of immunohistochemical stains, then there's about a 30 to 40% chance that other lymph glands are involved. It's important in this case to organize more surgery or sometimes radiation therapy.

The prospect of facing more surgery is very frustrating and may feel like another hill you have to climb, but hang in there. The good news is that your treatment team has found the exact location of the cancer cells and will now tailor the best treatment plan for your particular circumstances.

CONTROL POINT #12 – DO I NEED MORE SURGERY?

WARNING

If a sentinel node is definitely involved, and particularly if a pathologist can see the cancer cells without the assistance of immunohistochemical stains, then there's about a four in ten chance that other lymph glands are involved in your armpit.

TIP

After breast conservation, 2 mm margins are ideal but we sometimes accept tighter margins depending on the circumstances, particularly when you have follow-up radiation therapy.

REMEMBER

The two important parts of your pathology report that determine the need for more surgery are whether or not the margins of excision are clear and whether or not cancer cells are found in your sentinel node.

CONTROL POINT #13

WHAT DOES MY PATHOLOGY REPORT REALLY MEAN?

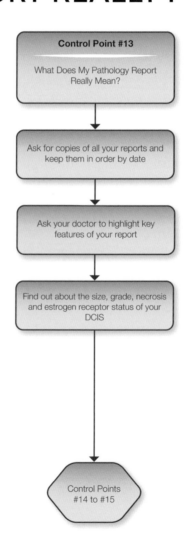

Control Point #13

What Does My Pathology Report Really Mean?

↓

Ask for copies of all your reports and keep them in order by date

↓

Ask your doctor to highlight key features of your report

↓

Find out about the size, grade, necrosis and estrogen receptor status of your DCIS

↓

Control Points #14 to #15

What Does My Pathology Report Really Mean?

The next step is for you and your doctor to understand your pathology report fully. The pathology report can be a bit scary—it's usually in very detailed medical language that may be difficult to understand. Some of my patients get frightened by reading some aspects of the report.

The pathology report looks at your DCIS (what we called a "weed" in the garden example earlier) in very fine detail. It described not only what the "weed" looks like when you view it with the naked eye (the macroscopic report), but also what its real structure looks like under the microscope (the **microscopic report**) (Figure 13.1). The pathologist works out whether it's a weed that can spread its seed to other parts of the garden (that is, it is not DCIS but invasive breast cancer), or one that is indeed DCIS as was determined by your core biopsy and will remain localized in the same garden patch or the breast. On the next few pages, I list what needs to be recorded in a good "formatted" or "structured"

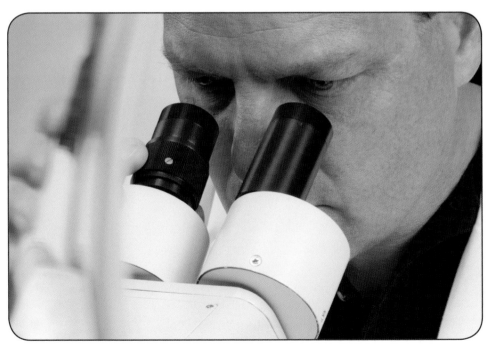

Figure 13.1 It can take more than a week for a final pathology report.

report. This is essentially a checklist of what the pathologist should document in his report and is now included in many international guidelines.

Many pathologists still use a paraphrased report, which is a long narrative. I find these quite difficult to read, and important information is sometimes not clearly stated or omitted. The structured report, on the other hand, allows the oncologist to find the important elements (or factors) in your pathology quickly, and it also highlights the important aspects of the report to you.

We are trying to understand the specifics about your DCIS by reading the pathology report and:

- ensuring that there are no invasive areas with your DCIS or cells in the sentinel node, in which case it is not a pure DCIS

- checking that the DCIS has been removed with clear margins

- looking for factors that may increase the chance of DCIS or invasive cancer coming back in the same or opposite breast.

Do remember, however, that the pathology report is only an indication. There is always hope and it's important for you to do what you can to take some control. Understand your report, but don't get too overwhelmed if there are a few negative findings. Usually, there are positive findings as well.

The pathology report is complicated. Ask for a photocopy of it. It is your breast and your breast tumor, and you really need to know what's going on. Be polite but firm. There are two parts to the pathology report. As mentioned, the first section is called the macroscopic report and the second section is called the microscopic report. Further tests are conducted in the pathology lab on your DCIS to work out whether it is likely to respond to hormonal treatments and to ensure that the sentinel node is totally clear. These extra tests take longer than the routine testing and often two or three amended or supplementary reports are issued after your original report.

Understanding the Macroscopic Report

The macroscopic report addresses what can be seen with the naked eye. It's not usually done by the specialist pathologist, but perhaps by his assistant, such as a resident in training. Parts of it may be documented by a technician.

The macroscopic report includes:

- The type of specimen (a breast conservation specimen or a mastectomy specimen).

- Information about any scars on the skin or if the nipple has been removed.

- The dimensions (and usually the weight) of the excised specimen.

- The dimensions of the macroscopic tumor. In other words, if they can see an abnormality that looks like a cancer, they may measure it at this point. This is usually measured in millimeters or centimeters, but sometimes inches. Usually there is no visible lump, but the breast tissue may look different. Comedo carcinoma involving multiple ducts occasionally produces a firm mass. If DCIS presents as a lump then it can appear as a well-defined, tan tumor to the naked eye. Earlier, I mentioned that the name comedo was derived from the white to pale yellow which can be squeezed out from the cut surface. Abundant calcification in the lesion can impart a gritty sensation upon cutting into the tumor. Although these findings are suggestive of comedo DCIS, an identical gross appearance is found in benign tumors or even mastitis.

- The distance between the tumor and the cut edge of the specimen (the macroscopic margin).

- The presence of any other abnormalities, such as a second unsuspected or previously discovered cancer.

- An indication of which parts or sections of the specimen (called "blocks") have been sampled.

- The handling protocol that was used. Surgeons may use different techniques to identify the orientation of specimen for the pathologist. One convention is to place a short stitch on the superior (head side) of the excised specimen, a long stitch on the lateral (or armpit side) of the specimen, and a medium-length stitch on the medial (breast bone side) of your specimen.

The lab will ink the outside of your specimen when it receives it so they can see where the surgeon's margin is located under the microscope. After the specimen is inked and dried it will be sliced into thin, usually 4 mm or so, slices or "sections". Sometimes these slices are also X-rayed to guide the pathologist to the actual area of any microcalcifications originally seen on your mammogram.

The combination of the sutures and the inking allows the pathologist to orient your specimen a shown in Figure 13.2. The various, internationally defined margins are:

- medial which is the cut edge near your breastbone

- lateral which is the one toward your armpit

- anterior shown on the right side of Figure 13.2 which shows what happens when you take out a slice and lay it flat. This is the margin toward the skin of your breast

- posterior which is the margin toward your ribs and muscles

- superior is the one toward your head

- inferior is the one toward your feet.

In Figure 13.2, the "closest margin" is the anterior margin. If a margin is involved or too close, knowing these directions can help the surgeon take an extra shave, or "re-excision," in that particular direction.

For smaller specimens, under about 30 mm, every single slice is examined under the microscope. For larger specimens, including mastectomy specimens, it is impossible to examine every single slice, and the sampling and examination technique will vary. Sometimes we ask the pathologist to examine more or "deeper" blocks if something doesn't quite add up. For all specimens, however, the extreme edges are always examined to ensure that the size is accurately determined. In Figure 13.2, if we assume the DCIS extends over three sections (of 4 mm) then the length of the DCIS can be estimated to be 12 mm or 1.2 cm.

I use a lot of the information above to work out how much normal tissue the surgeon has removed compared to the size of the breast tumor, and to calculate how close the DCIS is to the edge of the specimen. The microscopic report gives us more detail about the nitty-gritty of your DCIS.

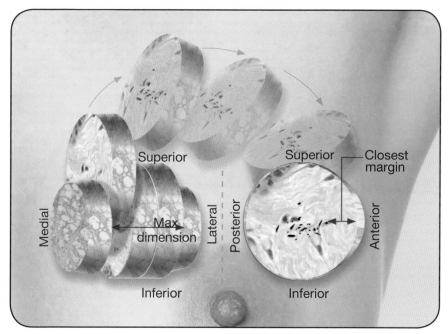

Figure 13.2 Once the area containing your DCIS is removed from your breast it is divided into 4 mm slices and the pathologist studies how close it is to the various margins shown and documents the closest margin. The lateral margin is toward your armpit and the medial toward your breastbone.

Understanding the Microscopic Report

The section below is quite detailed and you may want to skip part or all of it. The following are what I look for in the microscopic report.

Type of Procedure

Confirm that breast conservation or mastectomy was done (this is sometimes only recorded at the top of the report in the macroscopic section). If it was a mastectomy, was it a skin-sparing or nipple-sparing mastectomy?

Tumor Site or Location

It's important to correlate what is seen on the pathology report with what was seen on the preoperative mammogram or ultrasound and also with where you felt a breast lump if one was present. Some pathologists go to the trouble of documenting the location of the tumor, but usually in terms of a quadrant (or a quarter of the breast). The most common location is the upper outer quadrant, which is the quarter toward the armpit (as shown earlier in Figure 4.2 on page 59).

Tumor Type

This is a summary of the different types of DCIS that I mentioned in "Control Point #1 – What on Earth Is DCIS?" (Figures 1.2–1.5 on page 20). There can be overlap, and the reality is that it can be difficult to classify one type of DCIS as fitting neatly into one category. There are often mixtures of architecture as well as grade. As mentioned, for DCIS, we not only look at the architecture or pattern, but we also look at other factors such as nuclear grade and necrosis (which I will discuss below). Common tumor types include: comedo, solid, cribriform, and papillary/micropapillary. Uncommon patterns include: clinging, apocrine, encysted papillary, clear cell, signet ring, neuroendocrine, and cystic hypersecretory. I do find the type of DCIS helps me correlate it with the mammographic findings. As noted in "Control Point #1 – What on Earth Is DCIS?," there is better correlation between the area of microcalcification on a mammogram and the comedo, or solid subtypes, of DCIS. We also know that papillary DCIS can be quite a widespread process in some, but not all, patients. Encysted papillary DCIS is uncommon, tends to occur in older women, and is usually confined to the capsule of the cysts without surrounding DCIS or areas of invasion; it may be a good subtype to observe after wide excision (particularly if the patient has other illnesses).

Pathologic Size of the Tumor

Most pathologists measure a tumor in three dimensions. For example, a tumor might be 20 mm × 10 mm × 10 mm. Sometimes a second area of DCIS or focus is mentioned, and in a good report, the distance between the two foci, or spots of DCIS, is documented. However, the truth is that size can be difficult to measure and is often deduced from counting the number of sections which contain DCIS and multiplying this by the slice thickness. This measures the length and then the largest width can also be measured. Basically as an oncologist, we try and put it all together by correlating the mammographic size with the pathology size and, more importantly, looking at the margins of resection as well.

Margins of Resection

This is quite a controversial area. No pathologist can really hold their hand on their heart and say that a margin is truly negative or positive. The first problem is that the pathologist can only report on what's been removed. As can be seen in "Brenda's Story" ("Control Point #15 – Do I Need Additional Tests?"), the margins were clear once her nipple area was removed due to Paget's disease, but the MRI scan and subsequent mastectomy revealed a further 7 cm area of high-grade DCIS and areas of microinvasion. The distance between the edge of the DCIS and the cut surgical edge can be measured using a scale visible to the pathologist using a calibrated eyepiece on a microscope.

Nuclear Grade

For patients with DCIS, we don't talk about **histologic grade** as we do for patients with invasive cancer. We do, however, document the nuclear grade of the DCIS, which refers to how abnormal the nucleus (or control center) of the cancer cell looks. This is scored in a range as low, intermediate or high grade. For the nuclear grade, the pathologist looks at the size of the nucleus, its shape, and its staining intensity, which helps to determine how much DNA content it has and whether it's highly abnormal (high grade) or closer to a normal cell (low grade). A high-power lens (40x) is used by the pathologist to compare the size of the tumor cells to that of normal cells and the size of a red blood cell. Three categories are assigned:

- **High nuclear grade**: These cells tend to be very irregular and vary markedly in size and shape. This marked irregularity in pathology-speak is called "pleomorphism." There is often a prominent **nucleolus**, which is a rounded body inside the nucleus. There is normally one nucleolus in each nucleus, but in this type of high-grade DCIS there is often more than one. The nucleus of the cell is often three or more times the size of red blood cells. Mitoses are often visible. **Mitosis** is where one cell divides into two cells and it is basically how DCIS can keep growing. The pathologist may say that "prominent mitoses are evident," meaning that he or she is more likely to call your DCIS a high-grade subtype. **Mitotic rate** is a measure taken into account when a tumor is graded; the pathologist counts how may cells dividing into two he or she can see in your tumor. High nuclear grade DCIS is often present in the comedo, solid, and even micropapillary or cribriform patterns (Figure 13.3, right).

- **Intermediate nuclear grade**: These cases may have some features of low- or high-grade DCIS. The nerve centers don't vary in size and shape as much as high-grade DCIS but lack the uniformity of low-grade DCIS. The growth pattern can be solid, cribriform, or micropapillary (Figure 13.3, center).

- **Low nuclear grade**: This type of DCIS has cells which all look the same. The pattern is often called "monotonous" or "monomorphic." The nerve centers of the cells tend to be small and are one and a half to two times the size of a normal red blood cell. There are only "occasional nucleoli," with few, if any, cells dividing or with mitoses. The cells are very ordered and often "polarized," which means the cells are lining up in one direction. The cells look like the boards of a white picket fence, all lined up in a row with equal gaps between the palings (Figure 13.3, left).

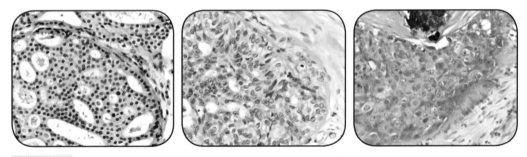

Figure 13.3 Low (left), intermediate (center), and high (right) nuclear grade DCIS.

Necrosis

This means death of cells. As mentioned earlier, when cells in the middle of a solid area of DCIS lose their blood supply, they essentially starve and then die off. This type of cell death is often called **comedonecrosis**. This type of necrosis has been found in some studies to be an indicator of a higher recurrence rate in the breast, particularly if radiation isn't given. Necrosis is more often seen in high-grade DCIS but can also be seen in all types of DCIS. Necrosis can also occur in individual cells where it is considered to be less important than extensive areas of necrosis. Extensive necrosis implies high cell turnover, a stressed "microenvironment," which increases the chance of the cancer coming back if it is not treated effectively

Calcification

A good report should also mention whether or not there is calcification visible. In "Brenda's Story" ("Control Point #15 – Do I Need Additional Tests?"), the patient presented with Paget's disease of the nipple. There was no visible microcalcification on the mammogram, but the subsequent disease found on her MRI scan was found to be high-grade DCIS with areas of microcalcification. This is because microcalcification—when it is less than 100 microns—cannot be seen with the naked eye. When microcalcifications are recorded, it is also good to know if the calcium is:

- Necrosis associated: Areas of comedonecrosis are shut down by the body by depositing calcium in the area. This is what causes the worrying casting or linear microcalcifications described in "Control Point #1 – What on Earth Is DCIS?"

- Secretory type: These calcifications tend to cause distinct patterns—crystal-like ("crystalline"), layered ("laminated" or psammomatous type), or bone-like ("ossifying") and are usually associated with low-grade DCIS.

- Within benign elements: Calcifications, initially visible on your mammogram, may simply be associated with benign changes in your breast. A not uncommon benign area is called sclerosing adenosis, which starts off as an abnormality of the lobules. So if this is present, some of the micro-calcifications visible on your mammogram may have nothing to do with your DCIS. This may need to be taken into account when trying to work out how large is your area of DCIS and how to follow up with mammograms after your treatment. Some would argue that, in this setting, you may be better off with a mastectomy as follow-up would be difficult; whereas others would argue that as long as everyone knows the visible calcium spots are in areas of benign disease, follow-up could still involve regular mammograms looking for new or changing areas of calcium spots on your mammogram. MRI scanning may also help in this setting, and a new baseline MRI may help.

Calcium spots are usually the "front door" of DCIS. They help us detect the abnormal area in your breast. The challenge, as noted in "Control Point #1 – What on Earth Is DCIS?," is to work out what it really means. Is the calcified area DCIS or is it benign? If it is DCIS, then there are usually areas of DCIS that are not calcified as well. These are in areas closer to the duct's blood supply so that the abnormal cells have not died, nor have they undergone necrosis nor "repaired" with calcium.

Calcifications with distinctive crystalline, ossifying, and laminated appearances tend to occur in the step before DCIS as well (hyperplasia), which can lead to its detection on a mammogram. Patients with a type of hyperplasia called **columnar cell hyperplasia** may have other pathology present, and, hence, often it is worth going back and excising the area. It is beyond the scope of this book to go into too much more detail but, suffice it to say, if your biopsy has shown various types of hyperplasia with atypia, it may be best to excise the surrounding area. Over the years the terminology used has changed but may include terms like: CAPSS with atypia, where CAPSS indicates columnar alteration with prominent apical snouts and secretions; flat epithelial atypia (FEA); or columnar cell lesions (CCLs). In a review article, about one-third to one-quarter of patients with FEA seen at core biopsy were found to have a more advanced lesion at excision such as low-grade DCIS (Pandey et al. 2007). This could include tubular carcinoma, lobular carcinoma in situ, and **invasive lobular carcinoma**, as well as micropapillary DCIS. However, the jury is still out on these lesions and more research is required to work out the true level of an associated future DCIS or invasive cancer (Aroner et al. 2010).

Microinvasion—Present or Absent

A very important but often difficult condition to diagnose is the presence of DCIS just poking through the wall of the duct. This is called "microinvasion." This is often present in the setting of a large area of DCIS with one or more clearly separate areas of spread or "infiltration" into the surrounding tissue called the stroma, or supporting tissue surrounding the ducts (Figure 13.4). By definition, none of these areas measure more than 1 mm in diameter. If they are larger than this, then what you have is an actual breast cancer with surrounding DCIS.

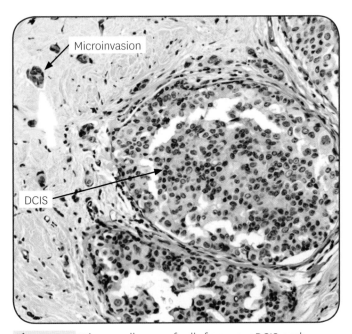

Microinvasion is rare if you do not have DCIS that is high nuclear grade. Cases of pure high or intermediate nuclear grade DCIS and those with comedo type necrosis are usually extensively sampled to exclude areas of invasion. One tricky area is when DCIS spreads "backwards" up the duct rather than down the duct into the lobules. This is called cancerization of lobules and can sometimes be mistaken for microinvasion. The pathologist uses a couple of tactics to help here. He or she may take deeper sections using standard stains or may use special immuno-histochemical stains.

Figure 13.4 When small areas of cells from your DCIS push through the surrounding duct into the surrounding area this is called microinvasion (arrowed).

Axillary Lymph Gland Involvement

As mentioned in "Control Point #5 – What Will I Do about My Armpit?," there are some situations where a sentinel node biopsy (or if not available, a sample of some of the lower axillary lymph nodes) may be worthwhile. The main indication is large areas of high-grade DCIS, measuring over 4 or 5 cm on the preoperative mammogram. Sometimes in this setting, the pathologist may find microinvasion as noted above, but this can sometimes be like looking for a needle in a haystack. Another way of assessing the possibility of unsuspected invasion is by checking the glands or lymph nodes draining the breast area. If you are having a mastectomy, a sentinel node biopsy may avoid the problem of finding unsuspected invasive cancer in a large area of DCIS and then having to go back and having a delayed axillary dissection. If you have only had a wide local excision, it is still possible to have a sentinel node procedure as part of a planned second operation of your axilla if invasion was found.

There is no doubt that it is the best to be node-negative if an axillary node has been sampled. Isolated tumor cells (ITCs) may be present. ITCs are defined as single tumor cells or small cell clusters not larger than 0.2 mm that are usually detected only by immunohistochemical (IHC) or molecular methods, but they may also be verified by the naked eye using purple stains (Figure 5.5 on page 77) known as hematoloxylin and eosin (H&E) stains. As mentioned earlier, there is a lot of controversy about what to do if a pathologist finds ITCs as part of his or her workup of the sentinel node. One area of controversy is whether the cells were simply dislodged at the time of your core biopsy or surgery and are simply trapped in the gland but are not biologically important. In other words, this is what we call a false positive due to passive transport of the cells.

However, there is a very small chance that after an initial diagnosis of pure DCIS additional areas of invasive disease may give axillary metastases. These areas can be missed due to sampling errors at the initial core needle biopsy or even after definitive breast surgery. The incidence of nodal invasion for patients with DCIS is less than 1% and similarly low (< 5%) in patients with DCIS with micro-invasion (van la Parra 2008).

If you are in this situation, don't panic because your prognosis is still very good. If you just have ITCs, we normally watch the armpit particularly if you are having radiation to the breast. If the disease in your gland is larger than an ITC, then further treatment should be considered such as an axillary sample or even hormonal treatment or chemotherapy in some circumstances. There is no one correct answer in this situation, so please talk to your treatment team about their own hospital policy.

The Estrogen Receptor

A detailed analysis of **estrogen-receptor (ER)** immunohistochemistry was provided by Bur et al. (1992). They classified 80% of 100 women with DCIS as being estrogen-receptor positive. There was a much higher frequency of receptor positivity in non-comedo (91%) than in comedo (57%) lesions. The frequencies of estrogen-receptor positivity among variants of non-comedo intraductal carcinoma did not differ significantly (cribriform, 89%; solid, 94%; micropapillary-papillary, 100%). These authors also confirmed the observation that estrogen-receptor status was almost always the same in the DCIS as any invasive parts of a lesion. This is important when evaluating a situation when you only have microinvasive disease where it is hard to get an adequate sample to test for ER status.

Estrogen receptors look for **estrogen**; and when they bind with the estrogen, it generates a sequence of chemical changes that activate the cell. The association between hormone replacement therapy (HRT) and an increased risk of breast cancer is thought to be due to HRT "feeding" a preexistent cancer cell with estrogen, which can make it grow. It's a bit like giving fertilizer to a weed.

Theoretically, ER-positive cells may grow with estrogen produced by your body. Estrogen can be produced even after menopause. In younger women, it is produced by the ovaries and in muscle, fat, and adrenal glands (which produce androgens and enzymes that control your blood pressure and are located above the kidneys).

The HER2 Receptor

The **HER2 receptor** is present in all the cells in your body. The problem is that in one in five patients with an invasive breast cancer, part of the HER2 receptor has gone a little bit crazy and becomes "over-expressed." The HER2 receptor controls cell growth, and patients with HER2-positive tumors may have DCIS that is more aggressive because it divides more rapidly. The study of HER2 receptors for DCIS is less advanced than that of invasive breast cancer. In fact, women with high-grade DCIS have a much higher rate of HER2 positivity than women with invasive breast cancer.

There are two different ways that we measure the HER2 receptor. The quick test is performed with immunohistochemistry and is the most commonly used test. It's measured by a scoring system of 1, 2, or 3. The other type of testing is called an **ISH (in-situ hybridization)** test, which is more accurate but takes a week or two for the results.

Ho et al. (2000) found significantly higher frequencies of HER2 amplification in comedo than in non-comedo DCIS (69% versus 18%) and for high rather than low nuclear grade DCIS (63% versus 14%). Micropapillary and cribriform DCIS are usually HER2 negative.

CONTROL POINT #13 – WHAT DOES MY PATHOLOGY REPORT REALLY MEAN?

WARNING
The pathology report can be a bit scary. It's usually in very detailed medical language that may not make sense. Ask for a copy and ask your doctors to explain and highlight the key points.

TIP
Important parts of your report include the size, nuclear grade, margins, estrogen receptor status, and type of DCIS.

REMEMBER
DCIS is very curable. Understand your pathology report, but don't get too overwhelmed if there are a few negative findings. Usually, there are positive findings as well.

Hanna's Story

Hanna was aged 51 when she was discovered to have a 45 mm area of microcalcifications in her right breast after a screening mammogram. A core biopsy showed DCIS alone. As is our policy, we gave Hanna all the surgical options in an objective way including a wide local excision or a mastectomy.

We also advised that a sentinel node should be considered. The pathology showed an intermediate-grade area of DCIS with fourteen cells in the sentinel node. Despite a thorough review of the breast area, the pathologist could not find any areas of frank invasive cancer or any areas suspicious of microinvasion. The DCIS showed signs of estrogen sensitivity (called ER-positive).

We decided to treat her breast with radiation, making sure we covered the level I axillary lymph nodes with radiation and some tamoxifen.

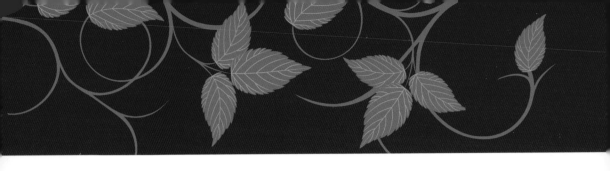

CONTROL POINT #14

WHAT IS MY PROGNOSIS?

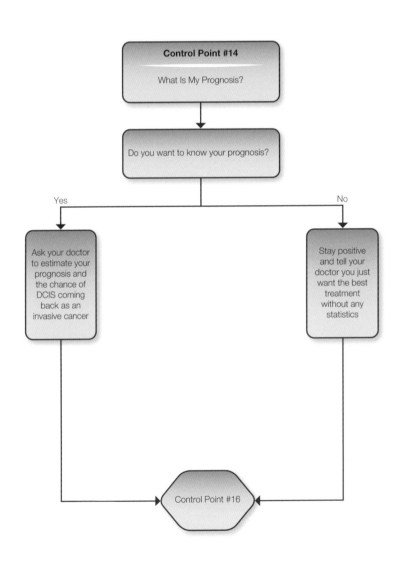

Control Point #14

What Is My Prognosis?

Do you want to know your prognosis?

Yes

No

Ask your doctor to estimate your prognosis and the chance of DCIS coming back as an invasive cancer

Stay positive and tell your doctor you just want the best treatment without any statistics

Control Point #16

Cure Rates Are Very High after Treatment of DCIS

The first thing to reassure you about is that your prognosis is *very, very* good after a diagnosis of DCIS. Usually if you have pure DCIS, the prognosis approaches 100%. I would like to apologize in advance, as this chapter is very mathematical. If you don't want to read all the detail right now, browse down to the next series of bullet points where I summarize the key facts. The reality is that it's never 100% because of two main factors:

1. the chance of dying of something else, like old age; or

2. the slightly higher chance of being diagnosed with breast cancer in your other breast.

So it is important when you are talking about how much therapy you need to always look at your life expectancy without DCIS. Table 14.1 shows the latest life expectancy figures.

Table 14.1 Average life expectancy (U.S., All races, from Arias 2010)

Current Age	Life Expectancy (Years)
30	+51
40	+42
50	+33
60	+24
70	+16
80	+9
90	+5

The table shows that if you are aged 80 you still, on average, have another nine years to live. That's a long time and you don't want to be bothered with DCIS coming back when you are 89! You may wish to just have your breast removed which is almost a 99% guarantee that it will never come back and all you will need is a check of the other breast from time to time. Or, depending on your life situation, you may say that you have ten years to go and you may want to be treated with breast conservation and minimize the chance of the DCIS coming back by having additional radiation therapy after your lumpectomy.

In fact, the meta-analysis of trials by the Early Breast Cancer Trialists' Collaborative Group (EBCTCG), who reviewed the outcome of the four largest trials in the world, found a ten-year risk of dying from breast cancer of 4.1% after conservative surgery and radiation and 3.7% after conservative surgery alone. However, this includes women who subsequently developed an invasive cancer on the other side so it's a little hard to tease out whether a new cancer in the other breast or a recurrent cancer on the treated side was the culprit in this analysis (EBCTCG 2010).

Fifteen-year results have now been published from the large European trial (EORTC 10853) which compared conservative surgery with or without radiation for DCIS. The 15-year risk of a DCIS recurrence after a local excision without radiation was 16%, which was halved to 8% by the addition of radiation. For an invasive recurrence, the corresponding rates were 16% and 10%. This study, like most studies of DCIS, was never large enough to pick up such small differences in cure rates. The 15-year chance of being free of breast cancer in another part of the body was 96% and 95% with or without radiation after a lumpectomy (Donker et al. 2013).

The large U.S. trials also tried to look at the risk of developing incurable **metastatic disease**, spreading to another part of the body from an invasive breast cancer recurrence, after a previous diagnosis of DCIS. In the B-17 trial, which compared lumpectomy with or without radiation, there was no difference in the risk of dying between the two groups. Deaths attributed to breast cancer were very uncommon and were 3.1% after lumpectomy alone, 2.7% (B-24 trial) to 4.7% (B-17 trial) after lumpectomy and radiation, and 2.3% after lumpectomy and radiation and tamoxifen (Wapnir et al. 2011).

It is too early to tell for sure if the addition of tamoxifen is causing a real reduction in the chance of dying of a future breast cancer or not. Similarly, it is hard to tease out the contribution to the statistics of breast cancer appearing on the other side (Stuart et al. 2011). I suspect a lot of the benefit is from reducing the risk of invasive cancer on either side, but ultimately, the difference with and without tamoxifen at ten years is in the order of 1% to 2% so this must be carefully balanced with your current age and general condition and the side-effects of tamoxifen. The cost-benefit ratio is probably better for women diagnosed with DCIS under the age of 50, who have a lot longer to live and therefore more time for a recurrence to occur in the same breast or opposite breast. I will discuss this further in "Control Point #17 – Do I Need Hormonal Treatment?".

One long-held theory is that radiation on one side can increase the risk of breast cancer on the other side. However in the B-17 trial, the actual incidence of opposite breast cancer at fifteen years was no different whether radiation was given or not. The risk of developing breast cancer on the other side was one in ten over a fifteen-year period. Basically, not a very high risk. About two-thirds of tumors in the other breast were invasive breast cancer and one-third was DCIS. When tamoxifen was added (in the NSABP B-24 trial), the risk of breast cancer developing in the opposite healthy side was 7.3% at fifteen years compared to 10.8% if no tamoxifen was given. So a lot of the benefit is in tamoxifen preventing cancer developing on the other side, whereas, radiation works well on the affected side. There will be more on this in "Control Point #17 – Do I Need Hormonal Treatment?".

The NSABP group also examined the risk of dying from breast cancer if a woman developed an invasive breast cancer recurrence. There were thirty-nine deaths among the 263 women with an invasive breast cancer recurrence on the same side. The risk of dying from breast cancer after treated DCIS recurred as an invasive breast cancer on the affected side was 10% at ten years (Wapnir et al. 2011). The European study, however, showed that although there was no increased risk of dying from breast cancer when DCIS recurred in the breast, 40% of patients died by 20-years after an invasive recurrence

(Donker et al. 2013). This difference of 10% for the U.S. study and 40% in the European study cannot be explained easily but needless to say, preventing a more serious invasive recurrence is one of the benefits of having radiation.

In the UK/ANZ (U.K., Australia, and New Zealand) trial, only thirty-nine of 1,694 women (2%) died of breast cancer, and the outcome was not different based on whether or not radiation or tamoxifen was given after conservative surgery.

So what can we make of all this mass of potentially confusing information?

- The chance of being cured after a diagnosis of DCIS is probably 98 to 99%.

- Once you have DCIS on one side, there is a small increase in the risk of invasive breast cancer or DCIS on the other side, thus requiring an annual mammogram for follow-up.

- If DCIS recurs as an invasive breast cancer on the same side, then the ten-year subsequent cure rate is 90% (U.S. study) but as low as 60% 20 years later (European study).

- It is, therefore, important to keep the invasive recurrence rate as low as possible.

- Tamoxifen may be important, particularly in reducing the risk of breast cancer in your other side, but it only helps a little and in "Control Point 17 – Do I Need Hormonal Treatment?" I will look into the cost and benefits of taking tamoxifen.

What Determines DCIS or Invasive Cancer Coming Back after Treatment?

Table 14.2 on page 155 shows the risk of a recurrence in your breast after conservative surgery or conservative surgery and radiation therapy. In this next section, I will try to tease out the risk factors for you using the data from the Early Breast Cancer Trialists' Collaborative Group (EBCTCG), which examined a total of 3,729 women who participated in four clinical trials comparing radiation or observation after breast conserving surgery.

The evidence shows that we can reduce the chance of anything coming back in the breast quite a lot by adding radiation. In the last column of table 14.2, I have calculated the percentage reduction in recurrence, which ranged from 23 to 67%. On average, radiation reduced the risk of a recurrence in the breast by about half.

Patient Factors

Patient factors predicting recurrence in the breast include younger age at diagnosis and the presence of a family history of breast cancer. Younger age has been associated with a higher risk of a recurrence in the breast, particularly if you are less than forty years of age at diagnosis. The reasons for this association are not entirely clear, although one study found that younger women (which they defined as being under forty-five years of age at diagnosis) had more higher-grade tumors (nearly 70%) as the main contributing factor (Goldstein et al. 2000).

Some, but not all, studies have found that having a family history of breast cancer is associated with a higher risk of DCIS or invasive cancer coming back after breast conservation. In a small study from

New Orleans, women with a family history who did not have radiation after a lumpectomy had a recurrence rate in the breast of 10% compared to 2% for those without a family history. For women who had a mastectomy or radiation after a lumpectomy, family history did not increase the risk of a recurrence. In other words, if you have a family history of breast cancer, it is probably best to have something more than just a lumpectomy for your DCIS (Szelei-Stevens, 2000).

Tumor Factors

Factors that predict a higher recurrence, particularly if radiation is not given, include if your DCIS is over 20 mm, if it is high-grade, and, more importantly, if it extends to the surgical margins or if it's in more than one part of the breast ("multifocal"). Involved margins predicted an increased risk of recurrence even after radiation. In order to look at several factors at the same time, the EBCTCG looked at patients with DCIS which was small (under 20 mm) with clear margins. Significantly, they found that the risk of recurrence was high for low-grade or high-grade DCIS. In the EBCTCG, the ten-year risk of recurrence was 30% without radiation and 12% with radiation for low-grade DCIS. For intermediate- to high-grade DCIS, the risk was 25% without radiation and 15% with radiation (EBCTCG 2010). In other words, just because something is low-grade does not mean that it can't come back. In fact, the data shows that the risk of recurrence is the same irrespective of grade. It is likely that small low-grade DCIS, under 10 mm, with clear margins will have a lower risk, but this was not reported in this study.

In the early 1990s, Eastern Cooperative Oncology Group (ECOG) designed a nonrandomized registration study (ECOG E5194) to attempt to identify suitable patients with DCIS for treatment using local excision alone (with omission of radiation treatment). The two arms of the study were: (1) low- or intermediate-grade DCIS, 2.5 cm in size or less or (2) high-grade DCIS, 1.0 cm in size or less. A minimum negative margin width of 3 mm was required. The protocol was amended in 2000 to allow the option to take adjuvant tamoxifen.

For patients entered into the ECOG E5194 study, the average size of the DCIS lesion was 6 mm and 5 mm in the two arms, respectively. With a median follow-up of 6.2 years for the 565 patients with low- or intermediate-grade DCIS, the five-year rate of **local recurrence** on the affected side was 6.1% and the seven-year rate was 10.5%. With an average follow-up of 6.7 years for the 105 patients with high-grade DCIS, the five-year rate of local recurrence was 15.3% and the seven-year rate was 18.0%. The authors advised that patients with high-grade DCIS are not suited for treatment with excision alone (without radiation) even when the DCIS area was small; but for patients with low- or intermediate-grade DCIS, additional follow-up would be needed to determine the long-term results as low-grade cancer can take a long time to return (Solin et al. 2010).

Treatment Factors

The EBCTCG also looked at whether the extent of surgery reduced the risk of recurrence and found that having more extensive conservative surgery was no better. Patients who had a "sector resection" (essentially removing the quadrant of the breast where the DCIS was located) had a recurrence rate in the breast of 30% compared to 27% where the DCIS was removed with a standard lumpectomy. On the other hand, tamoxifen reduced the risk of recurrence after a lumpectomy or lumpectomy and radiation.

Predicting Your Risk of Recurrence

You can work out your risk of a recurrence in the breast as in the following example. Assume Jean is aged 45, has a high-grade DCIS excised, and is considering avoiding radiation. The risk with one of those factors present is 29% if < 50 and 33% if high-grade. It's likely to be a little higher when both factors are present. So let's round it up to about 35%. Now make it 36% with no radiation, as it's easier to divide even numbers.

As a rule of thumb, radiation reduces the chance of a recurrence in the breast by half. That is, if it's 36% without radiation, it will be about 18% with radiation. Whatever the factor, nearly always half of the recurrences are invasive (shown in red in the graphs below) and half are DCIS (shown in orange). The actual figures from the table are: with radiation the risk is 18% if < 50 and 17% for high-grade.

Summary for Jean

Conservative Surgery Alone

Risk of DCIS recurrence: 18%

Risk of an invasive recurrence: 18%

Risk of dying of an invasive recurrence is a minimum 10%: $1/10^{th}$ of 18% is 1.8% (almost 2 in 100)

Conservative Surgery and Radiation

Risk of DCIS recurrence: 9%

Risk of an invasive recurrence: 9%

Risk of dying of an invasive recurrence is a minimum of 10%: $1/10^{th}$ of 9% is 0.9% (almost 1 in 100)

Now let's look at a situation which is of lower risk. Let's assume you have a type of low-grade DCIS that is small and you are in your 70s. Using the ECOG trial above, we can estimate that the risk of local recurrence may be around 12% at ten years without radiation.

Summary for Tanya

Conservative Surgery Alone

Risk of DCIS recurrence: 6%

Risk of an invasive recurrence: 6%

Risk of dying of an invasive recurrence is a minimum of 10%: $1/10^{th}$ of 6% is 0.6% (almost 6 in 1000)

Conservative Surgery and Radiation

Risk of DCIS recurrence: 3%

Risk of an invasive recurrence: 3%

Risk of dying of an invasive recurrence is a minimum of 10%: $1/10^{th}$ of 3% is 0.3% (almost 3 in 1000)

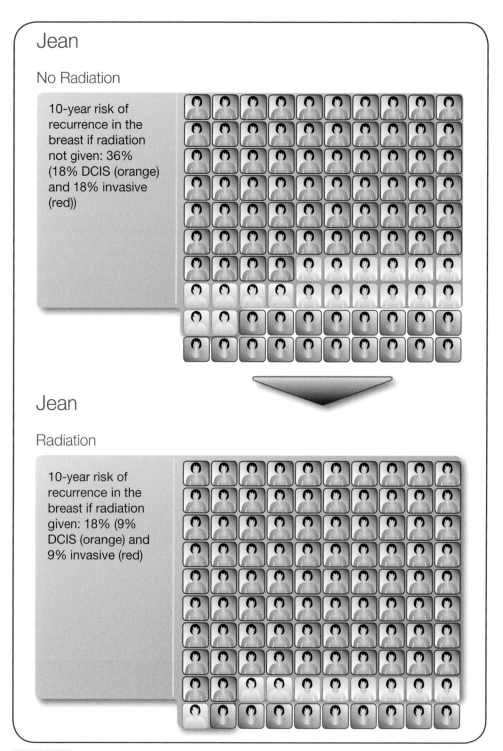

Figure 14.1 Jean is 45 years old with a 20 mm high-grade DCIS.

Tanya

No Radiation

10-year risk of recurrence in the breast if radiation not given: 12% (6% DCIS (orange) and 6% invasive (red))

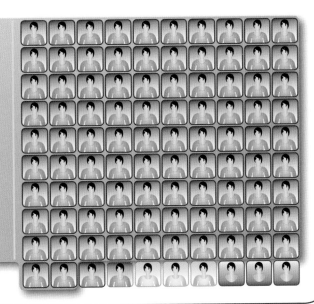

Tanya

Radiation

10-year risk of recurrence in the breast if radiation given: 6% (3% DCIS (orange) and 3% invasive (red))

Figure 14.2 Tanya is 70 years old with a 10 mm low-grade DCIS.

Another way of working out the risk of recurrence is using a calculator developed at the Memorial Sloan-Kettering Cancer Center. It is available at www.mskcc.org/APPLICATIONS/NOMOGRAMS/Breast/DuctalCarcinomaInSituRecurrencePage.aspx.

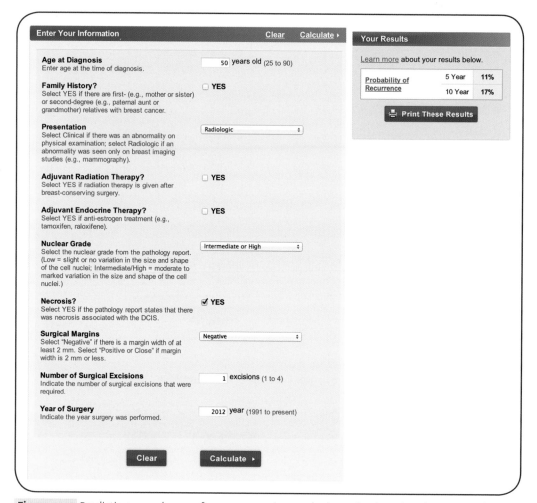

Figure 14.3 Predicting your chance of recurrence using a calculator developed at the Memorial Sloan-Kettering Cancer Center (input screen-left and results screen-right).

In the example shown in Figure 14.3, I have selected a fifty-year-old woman with high-grade DCIS, necrosis, and clear margins, and I have shown the risk without radiation or tamoxifen. The ten-year risk of a recurrence was calculated to be 17%. None of this is an exact science, but table 14.2 and the Web-based calculator will at least give you some knowledge, and therefore control, about risks of the DCIS coming back in the future with and without additional treatment after your surgery. Just remember that "recurrence" includes an invasive recurrence (which is more serious) half of the time and DCIS (which is still very treatable) in the other half. Also remember that most recurrences are treatable. See "Control Point #19 – What Checks Do I Need After my Treatment?".

Table 14.2 Risk of recurrence in the breast with or without radiation therapy

	Conservative Surgery	Conservative Surgery & Radiotherapy	Risk Reduced by
PATIENT FACTORS			
Age			
< 50	29.1%	18.5%	36%
≥ 50	27.8%	10.8%	61%
TUMOR FACTORS			
Detection			
Mammography Detection	27.8%	11.2%	60%
Clinical Detection	32.6%	20.7%	37%
Pathological Size			
1–20 mm	28.9%	13.1%	55%
20–50 mm	39.0%	13.0%	67%
Margin			
Clear	26.0%	12.0%	54%
Involved	43.8%	24.2%	45%
Nuclear Grade			
Low	28.4%	12.3%	57%
Intermediate	29.8%	15.5%	48%
High	33.1%	17.3%	48%
Comedonecrosis			
Present	36.5%	16.6%	55%
Absent	25.2%	12.0%	52%
Architecture			
Comedo/Solid	36.5%	19.0%	23%
Other	28.0%	13.0%	32%
Focality			
Unifocal	28.5%	11.2%	61%
Multifocal	42.2%	17.3%	59%
TREATMENT FACTORS			
Local Excision	27.0%	12.5%	54%
Sector Resection	30.4%	13.7%	55%
No Tamoxifen	28.8%	13.2%	54%
Tamoxifen	18.3%	9.3%	49%

The Van Nuys Prognostic Index (VNPI)

Silverstein et al. (1995) proposed a classification for DCIS carcinoma based on nuclear grade (high or low-intermediate) and the presence or absence of necrosis as part of a prognostic index. Three prognostic categories resulting from consideration of these variables were as follows: Group 1, low-intermediate nuclear grade without necrosis; Group 2, low-intermediate nuclear grade with necrosis; and Group 3, high nuclear grade with or without necrosis. The **Van Nuys Prognostic Index (VNPI)** included margin status and tumor size as well as these histologic groups. Follow-up revealed a significant correlation between the VNPI and the risk of recurrence in the breast after conservation therapy. It was suggested that patients with low VNPI scores (4 to 6) could be treated with excision alone; patients with intermediate scores (7 to 9) would benefit from radiation; and patients with high scores (> 10) seem to be most suited for a total mastectomy. Unfortunately, this scoring system has never been validated by prospective studies and is based on a small, select sample of patients and is not generally used.

Oncotype DX Assay

Genotyping might help identify high-risk and low-risk patients, as it does for invasive disease. Through tumor genotyping, researchers can detect the genetic abnormalities that give rise to particular tumors. It is these mutations that appear to "drive" healthy cells to become tumor cells. Diverse cancers may share the same genetic abnormalities. Genomic Health has recently released the Oncotype DX Breast Cancer Assay for DCIS—which, they claim, can estimate the likelihood of local recurrence (DCIS or invasive carcinoma) at ten years (www.oncotypedx.com/en-US/Breast/PatientsCaregiversDCIS).

The test produces the DCIS Score result, a number between 0 and 100, and analyzes twelve genes. The first clinical results were presented at the San Antonio Breast Conference in 2011 (Solin et al. 2011). The investigators used the gene test on pathology samples from the ECOG E5194 trial mentioned above. Of note, this was a very select group of patients where the average DCIS size was 7 mm and 97% were hormone-receptor positive and no patient received radiation. About one-third received tamoxifen. In this preliminary study, patients with a low DCIS score (< 39) had a recurrence rate of 12%; patients with an intermediate DCIS score (39–54) had a recurrence rate of 25%; and patients with high DCIS score (≥ 55) had a recurrence rate of 27%. The corresponding risk of invasive cancer recurrence was 5%, 9%, and 19% respectively. Its clinical applicability will become apparent only with time, particularly since, as I will show later, low-grade DCIS can take many years to progress.

So this is where it gets a little tricky. The dilemma is: Do we overtreat or potentially undertreat you in a situation where we can't look into the crystal ball and predict your future?

DCIS in Males

I have only seen two male patients with DCIS and both were elderly gentlemen who were treated by a total mastectomy. Interestingly, one male presented with a bloody nipple discharge and the other one had a lump. One of the largest series on DCIS in males comes from France. From 1970 to 1992, thirty-one cases of pure DCIS of the male breast treated in nineteen French Regional Cancer Center were reviewed (Cutuli et al. 1997).

They represented 5% of all breast cancers treated in men in the same period. The average age was fifty-eight years, but astonishingly, six patients were younger than forty years. In general, the age of occurrence for DCIS in men is younger than for invasive cancer, suggesting that DCIS is the first step in the development of breast cancer in men.

Twelve patients were discovered by a bloody nipple discharge and ten patients had a lump. Three patients (10%) had a family history of breast cancer. Six patients underwent lumpectomy, and twenty-five had a mastectomy.

Fifteen out of thirty-one lesions were of the papillary subtype, pure or associated with a cribriform component. The size of the twelve measured lesions varied from 3 to 45 mm. All lymph nodes sampled were negative. With an average follow-up of about seven years, four patients (13%) presented with a recurrence on the chest-wall at 12, 27, 36, and 55 months. Three of these four patients had been initially treated by a lumpectomy rather than a mastectomy. Radical salvage surgery was performed in three cases, but one patient developed metastases and died thirty months later. The last patient was treated by multiple local excisions and tamoxifen. This small study clearly shows to me that it is probably better for men to be treated by a mastectomy particularly as the impact on quality of life is far less dramatic than taking off a woman's breast.

CONTROL POINT #14 – WHAT IS MY PROGNOSIS?

WARNING

One of the biggest risk factors of DCIS coming back is whether or not the margins of resection are involved. Obtaining clear margins is an important goal of treatment.

TIP

For most people, the prognosis gets better with time. Sometimes we use a five-year figure because we know that if DCIS comes back, most of the time it comes back within five years. This is particularly the case with high-grade DCIS. Low-grade DCIS can come back a little slower and ten-year figures are better.

REMEMBER

Doctors can only give you a guide to your prognosis; they cannot predict your future with accuracy. In general, well-treated DCIS has a very good prognosis.

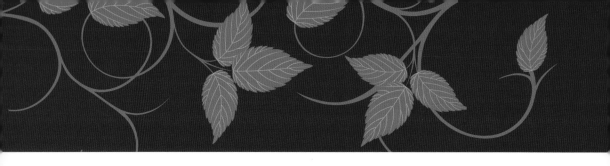

CONTROL POINT #15

DO I NEED ADDITIONAL TESTS?

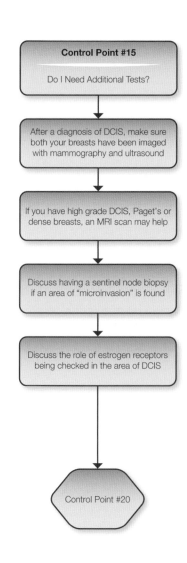

Control Point #15

Do I Need Additional Tests?

After a diagnosis of DCIS, make sure both your breasts have been imaged with mammography and ultrasound

If you have high grade DCIS, Paget's or dense breasts, an MRI scan may help

Discuss having a sentinel node biopsy if an area of "microinvasion" is found

Discuss the role of estrogen receptors being checked in the area of DCIS

Control Point #20

Lots of Tests Are Usually Unnecessary

Once you are diagnosed with DCIS, it is normally unnecessary to have lots and lots of tests as it does not spread to other parts of the body. Below is a checklist of tests that you may want to ensure have been done in your own situation.

Mammogram and Ultrasound

Once you are diagnosed with DCIS in the breast, make sure that your healthy breast and the remaining parts of your affected breast are imaged. The first thing to make sure is that both breasts have had a mammogram and an ultrasound. For example, very occasionally DCIS presents as a small lump. This may have been removed without any other imaging. You can still have a mammogram after this initial surgery. It's best to wait a couple of weeks as it will obviously hurt a little more in the already treated breast. If I have any concerns that the amount of breast tissue removed is smaller than the area of calcification I can see on the mammogram, a repeat mammogram may show residual tissue.

Breast MRI

In "Brenda's Story," the value of MRI if you have high-grade DCIS is clearly shown. Brenda had Paget's disease of the nipple removed with clear margins. However, we know from lots of publications that 93% of Paget's disease cases have underlying DCIS or invasive cancer. Brenda's MRI showed an area measuring 70 mm in the central part of the breast and another area measuring 20 mm in a different quadrant of the breast (Figure 1.12 on page 24). Both areas were located more than 5 cm from the nipple affected by Paget's disease. As mentioned in "Control Point # 8 – What Is Paget's Disease of the Nipple?", Paget's is often the tip of the iceberg. If you have Paget's or a dense breast on your mammogram or any other situation where your mammogram may not be accurate enough, an MRI of both breasts may be helpful (Figure 15.1). In Brenda's case, a mastectomy was the only way to remove all the abnormal area with clear margins.

In a good study from Nice, France, thirty-three patients with DCIS who had a core-biopsy-proven DCIS underwent a clinical examination, mammogram, and MRI and had the findings compared to the final pathology results. MRI detected 97% of the lesions. Lesion size was correctly estimated (± 5 mm), underestimated (< 5 mm), or overestimated (> 5 mm), respectively, by MRI in 60%, 19%, and 21% of cases and by mammography in 38%, 31%, and 31% of cases.

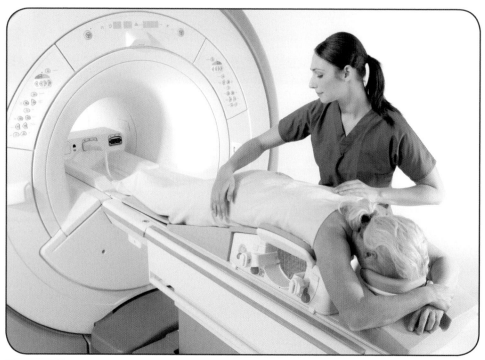

Figure 15.1 An MRI scan involves a tunnel type machine that uses magnetic fields to obtain an image of your breasts while lying face down. It also involves an injection of contrast into a vein.

If you do not have access to an MRI, don't worry as the study also found that the average size of each DCIS case was not too different for mammography versus MRI. This was 26 mm at histopathology, 28 mm at MRI, and 27 mm on mammography, which is not too far off. In another study from the University of Pennsylvania, for women with DCIS who received radiation, having an MRI did not change their prognosis compared to women who did not have an MRI (Solin et al. 2008). In contrast, a study from the University of Bonn in Germany found that MRI was far better at detecting DCIS than mammography. Of 167 women who had undergone both imaging tests preoperatively, only ninety-three (56%) were diagnosed by mammography and 153 (92%) by MRI (Kuhl et al. 2007). We are still learning about MRI and at this stage, I would not worry too much if you haven't had an MRI, particularly if your breasts are easy to view using a standard mammogram.

Additional Pathology Tests

Just because you have had your surgery doesn't mean the lab cannot do more tests on your breast specimen. At a minimum, make sure your surgeon does an estrogen receptor test on your specimen. I will explain this a bit more in "Control Point #17 – Do I Need Hormonal Treatment?".

In some situations where there is doubt about the presence of microinvasion, the pathologist can do markers of the various linings of the duct called keratin or myoepithelial markers. They can also cut into deeper levels of your breast specimen, which means they can study a larger area of your breast specimen carefully looking for any areas of microinvasion. If there is any microinvasion, a HER2 test may be helpful as it may determine the potential aggressiveness of the areas of invasion through the duct and the possible value of drugs like **Herceptin (trastuzumab)**. I am aware of one study at the moment recruiting patients with high-grade DCIS and testing them for HER2. If they are part of the 30% shown to be HER2-positive, then the patients are being offered, through allocation by a computer, two courses of Herceptin during their radiation or just radiation (Julian 2012).

Sentinel Node Mapping

As mentioned in "Control Point #5 – What Will I Do about My Armpit?," evaluation of your glands by a sentinel node may be useful if there is any hint of microinvasion around your DCIS. If you have true invasion (after, for example, a preoperative diagnosis of DCIS on core biopsy) then I would definitely recommend a sentinel node biopsy. Although not as accurate, it is still possible to do this test at this stage.

Tests for Others Parts of Your Body

Remember that DCIS does not spread to other parts of your body. Very rarely, we see a patient with high-grade DCIS that has spread to the lymph node. Despite looking at the DCIS in the breast we can't find any areas of microinvasion. This is because it's hard to sample every cubic centimeter of large areas of high-grade DCIS. If this has happened, you now have invasive breast cancer and you'd best get a copy of my first book, *Breast Cancer: Taking Control*. Most pains at the point of diagnosis are due to arthritis or muscular pains, and are not due to cancer. If a pain is persistent and does not go away with simple Tylenol (acetaminophen)/Panadol (paracetamol), then X-rays will be necessary.

CONTROL POINT #15 – DO I NEED ADDITIONAL TESTS?

WARNING Always make sure both your breasts have been imaged carefully. Sometime in the rush to get your involved breast looked at, the other side may not have yet had a breast ultrasound.

TIP If there is any concern that the area of microcalcifications on your original mammogram may not have been all removed, a repeat mammogram and/or MRI is still possible.

REMEMBER Check that your surgeon has performed an estrogen receptor test on your DCIS.

Brenda's Story

This diagnosis seemed a long time coming. I was 54 at the time and teaching in a small primary school at the base of the Blue Mountains west of Sydney. We had six children who were all teenagers and older. In early 2010, I first noticed a small amount of yellow discharge that resembled dry milk in the crevices of one nipple. At first I was able to rub it off. However, it reappeared days later, exposing a moist area underneath.

A visit to a local GP resulted in a mammogram, which came back negative, via a message from the surgery staff. That was a relief, and there was no call for any further follow-up.

Weeks passed and there was still no change in the nipple … but the secretion did not go away. So I went to another GP in the same practice who at first tried an antibiotic cream for two weeks. Seeing that this did not clear up the condition, he referred me to a dermatologist who took a biopsy of the surface of the nipple. This came back positive as Paget's disease.

I was then referred to a breast surgeon, who ordered both a mammogram and ultrasound. Both returned a clear report regarding any further indications of other cancers in the breast tissue.

Surgery to remove the nipple followed in early December of 2010. A second incision the following January, was needed to clear the margins and then it was off to radiation . . . or so I thought.

I was soon to graduate from a Master's degree program, and I wanted to attend the ceremony in Wagga Wagga. Knowing that this may delay the radiation treatment at my local hospital, I was offered the opportunity to have it sooner, at the hospital, where my surgery had taken place. We took that route and our first consultation resulted in the radiation specialist suggesting that I have an MRI. We did not hesitate and it was this test that revealed a large area of high-grade DCIS deep within the breast. Now, a full mastectomy was the only real option.

With that news came the need to decide on reconstruction or a straight mastectomy, and the decision needed to be made fairly smartly. That was difficult as, even though

I had a reasonable knowledge of the procedure, I had not had time to gather feedback from other women who were faced with the same decision. I decided to have reconstructive surgery at the same time as the mastectomy. This was now the third operation, called a skin-sparing mastectomy.

The results indicated that some of the DCIS had become microinvasive in quite a few areas. I was now dealing with invasive cancer which was also HER2 positive. I was on a rollercoaster, and a chemotherapy schedule began in order to reduce the risk of the cancer returning.

I have now completed the more intensive period of chemotherapy and Herceptin and look back with extreme gratitude for the encouragement to have the MRI. It dramatically changed the direction of my diagnosis and subsequent treatment.

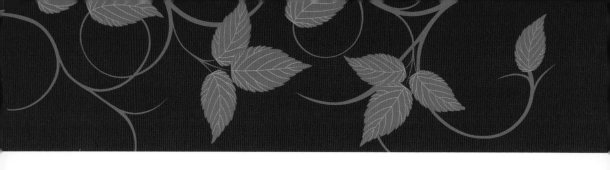

CONTROL POINT #16

DO I NEED RADIATION THERAPY?

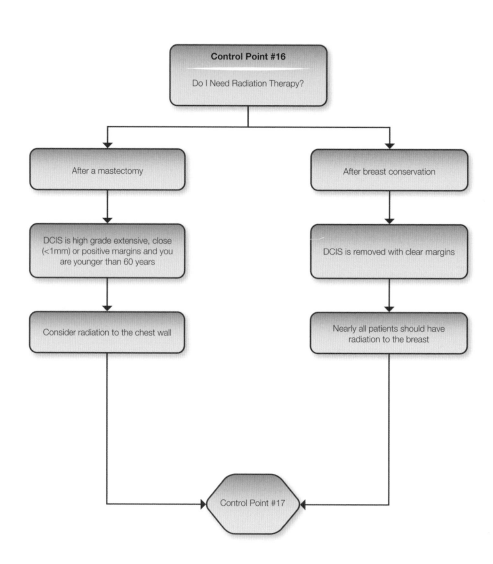

Control Point #16

Do I Need Radiation Therapy?

After a mastectomy

After breast conservation

DCIS is high grade extensive, close (<1mm) or positive margins and you are younger than 60 years

DCIS is removed with clear margins

Consider radiation to the chest wall

Nearly all patients should have radiation to the breast

Control Point #17

What Is Radiation Therapy?

There is no doubt that you may not really "hear" what the doctor is saying if you're suddenly hit with words like: "You now need radiation therapy." You may not even have been warned about this possibility before your surgery.

Radiation therapy basically uses X-rays to destroy cancer cells. There are many different forms of radiation, but the most common type used to treat women with breast cancer is what we call **external-beam radiation**. Radiation is produced when electrons are shot between a cathode (usually made of copper) and an anode (usually made of tungsten). Very soon after the discovery of radiation, it was found that it was able to destroy cancer cells because they're more sensitive to radiation than normal cells, such as your skin cells. When a small dose of radiation therapy is given every day for five to six weeks, the normal cells have a chance to recover, whereas the cancer cells do not have all the normal mechanisms to repair themselves.

Although radiation was first discovered in 1895, it was not routinely used for DCIS until the 1980s. The very first use of radiation after excision for DCIS was reported from the Institut Curie in France (Zafrani et al. 1986) and the MD Anderson Cancer Center in Texas, U.S.A. (Montague 1984). In each report, less than sixty patients with DCIS were treated with a wide excision and radiation and the early results were encouraging, which allowed other pioneers to follow in similar research. We have now proven that radiation is a very effective treatment following conservative surgery for DCIS.

Radiation therapy damages the DNA or genetic material of cells in the area being treated, stopping these cells from growing and dividing. Although radiation damages both DCIS cells and normal cells, most normal cells can recover within a few hours because they have all the repair mechanisms present to do so, whereas DCIS cells, because they are abnormal cells, can't repair themselves as well. Radiation given after surgery is called "adjuvant" radiation.

Radiation Therapy to the Whole Breast after Breast Conservation

A very common question I'm asked is: "Why do I need to have radiation to my breast after a lumpectomy when it's been removed by surgery?" This is a very good, logical question. For some reason, for many, but not all patients, surgery alone is not enough.

As mentioned earlier, if we look at my basic garden example, not giving radiotherapy to your breast after breast conservation surgery is like not putting a weed mat or straw mulch down after you remove a weed from under a rosebush in your garden. Even though the soil looks clear, some seeds may have been left behind, and the weed can come back again.

I won't go into too much detail on **partial breast irradiation (PBI)** except to say that it's best to do this if you're in a trial situation and will be closely monitored. Theoretically at least, not treating the whole breast will increase the risk of breast cancer coming back in other parts of the breast, but this could be a reasonable option if you're older, have a small area of low-grade DCIS that is well demarcated on a mammogram, surgically removed with a good margin, and if you have difficulty accessing five to six weeks of radiation. The American Society for Radiation Oncology (ASTRO) established a Task Force to review the evidence for and against PBI and categorized three groups of patients who may be eligible for PBI. The groups were classified as "acceptable" for PBI, "cautionary," and "unacceptable." Because of the limited trial data for women with DCIS, the ASTRO group did not include women with pure DCIS in the "acceptable" category.

The Task Force formed a consensus for the "cautionary" group, for whom "caution and concern in the use of PBI should be exercised at this point" (Smith et al. 2009). They recommended limiting this treatment to a trial setting and restricting this practice to patients with DCIS who:

- are aged 50 or older
- have DCIS that is up to 3 cm in size on the pathology report
- have DCIS located in one area (unifocal).

DCIS over 3 cm was considered unacceptable for PBI. In my view, caution is also required for DCIS that we know tends to be in multiple areas of the breast such as low-grade variants such as the papillary sub-type or DCIS which is difficult to detect on a follow-up mammogram because it is not calcified. A small study of 126 patients with DCIS (average size, 6 mm) has been published showing early good results but the follow-up, in my opinion, is too short (twenty-four months) to allow meaningful analysis (Israel et al. 2010).

In September 2009, the National Institutes of Health (NIH) consensus development and state-of-the-science conference about the diagnosis and treatment of DCIS noted:

> If radiotherapy is used, whole-breast radiotherapy is the standard technique, although accelerated partial-breast radiotherapy is being studied in ongoing clinical trials. Investigation of partial-breast radiotherapy and accelerated radiotherapy regimens is an appropriate focus of clinical research.

The full statement can be found here: http://consensus.nih.gov/2009/dcisstatement.htm

One of the most important breast conservation trials to date, performed by U.S. physician Bernard Fisher was for invasive breast cancer. When that trial was successful in showing that breast conservation was as effective as mastectomy for women with invasive disease, the next step was to test the usefulness of radiation after a lumpectomy for DCIS (Wapnir et al. 2011). Women with DCIS were enrolled in the NSABP B-17 trial between October 1985 and December 1990.

About 400 women had a lumpectomy only and 400 had lumpectomy and five weeks of radiation. The recurrence rates were:

- lumpectomy alone: 19% invasive and 16% DCIS (total 35%)

- lumpectomy and radiation: 9% invasive and 9% DCIS (total 18%).

It is important to note, however, that:

- Mammography was not as sophisticated as it is today and MRIs were not used.

- There was less understanding of the relationship of margins and the risk of a recurrence after breast conservation.

- Tumor receptors were not routinely performed.

- Hormonal treatments like tamoxifen were never given.

In other words, the fifteen-year results are likely to be a worst-case scenario. Taking this into account, it is likely that the chance of DCIS or invasive breast cancer coming back after radiation therapy to the breast is about 1% per year after radiation, reduced from about 2% per year after lumpectomy alone.

In the next chapter, I will look at the impact of tamoxifen in addition to a lumpectomy and/or radiation in the NSABP B-24 trial and a large trial from the U.K. and Australasia. As I will show, tamoxifen can have a small impact on reducing the risk of cancer coming back in the same breast, the opposite breast, and possibly, at least for a few women, in the rest of the body.

In October 2010, the Early Breast Cancer Trialists' Collaborative Group (EBCTCG) based at Oxford performed a meta-analysis where the data from four randomized trials comparing lumpectomy to lumpectomy and radiation therapy were combined. A total of 3,729 women were included in the study. Radiotherapy reduced the ten-year risk of any recurrence in the same breast by just over 15% (12.9% with radiation versus 28.1% without radiation). After ten years of follow-up, however, there was no significant effect on the risk of dying from invasive breast cancer (EBCTCG 2010).

Ultimately, what we're trying to do is to get rid of a small burden of tumor potentially left behind after a lumpectomy by the addition of radiation therapy. However, before you start thinking I'm unreasonable by recommending radiation for everyone, I always try to estimate the risk of recurrence with and without radiation. I look at the patient and see what else is going on in their lives, where they live, and if they are sick from other more serious conditions before I recommend a course of radiation. However, I am also aware that if you have lived to 80 years, then you have a chance of living another nine years or if you are 70 years old, you could live another 16 years on average (Arias 2010) (Table 14.1, on page 147). So don't let anybody say you are "too old" just because you are over 70! Sometimes it's better to deal with your condition with a short course of radiation now rather than waiting until you are older and perhaps frailer and less able to tolerate surgery for a DCIS which comes back.

Radiation Therapy after a Mastectomy

I have been treating patients with DCIS since the late 1980s and have only seen a handful of women who present with a new recurrence on their chest wall. The reason is that it is impossible for the surgeon to remove all the breast tissue after a mastectomy. Some surgeons use "thinner flaps" than others. Thinner flaps leave far less breast tissue behind. As mentioned earlier, it is also likely that the newer types of skin-sparing mastectomies may leave a little more normal breast tissue behind because of the complexity of the surgery, which has less access because of the use of smaller scars (Torresan et al. 2005). Taking control after a mastectomy means being vigilant about any new lumps or pimples that may appear on your skin over your chest. Most chest wall recurrences are in fact usually in the skin around your scar. In a meta-analysis, which I published back in 1999, we examined twenty-one older studies that treated 1,574 patients with a mastectomy following a diagnosis of DCIS. The chance of a chest wall recurrence was 1.4%. In fact, of the twenty-five patients whose disease recurred, nineteen (76%) came back as an invasive breast cancer (Boyages et al. 1999). In an update that we published, the risk increased to 3.3% at ten years (Stuart et al. 2011). I will talk about how to manage this situation later in "Control Point #19 – What Checks Do I Need after My Treatment?".

A recent study examined the risk of breast cancer coming back on the chest wall area with and without radiation. This study from California was based on eighty women who had a mastectomy for DCIS between 1994 and 2002 and did not receive radiation. Of the eighty patients, thirty-one had margins < 2 mm and forty-nine had margins of 2.1 to 10 mm. High-grade disease was observed in forty-seven patients; forty-five patients had comedonecrosis; and thirty had multifocal disease. Of the eighty patients, fifty-one were < 60 years of age. Of the thirty-one patients with a margin of less than 2 mm, five (16%) developed a recurrence on their chest wall versus only one of forty-nine patients (2%) with a margin of over 2 mm. Of the six patients with local recurrence, five had high-grade disease and/or comedonecrosis. All six recurrences were noted in patients < 60 years old. The authors suggest that those patients with margins under 2 mm, who are aged less than 60, or have high-grade disease, might benefit from post-mastectomy radiotherapy (Rashtian et al. 2008).

It's a tough call though, and it's best to discuss this with a radiation oncologist; and certainly close observation is probably a reasonable option in most situations. I find patients who are younger, who tend to have higher-grade DCIS, and who have the newer forms of mastectomy (skin-sparing and nipple-sparing) difficult to advise if their margins are clear but less than 2 mm. For example, giving radiation to the chest wall and the implant because the margin distance from the DCIS to the superficial skin is, say 0.5 mm, does increase the risk of hardening of the implant and possibly implant loss and may also lead to some skin changes. These concerns need to be balanced against the real risk of an invasive cancer or DCIS recurrence, particularly in and around the nipple region if that is left behind.

When and Where Is Radiation Therapy Given?

Radiation therapy usually starts between three to six weeks after surgery. This is provided that you can lift your arm above your head to get it out of the way and allow the radiation to target your breast or chest wall, and that all surgical wounds have healed. Normally, if hormonal drugs are given, we start these after the radiation is completed. The overall treatment options and strategy can be seen in Figure 16.1. If you have just had a lumpectomy, then radiation planning can take place as early as two weeks after your surgery and treatment can start three weeks after your surgery.

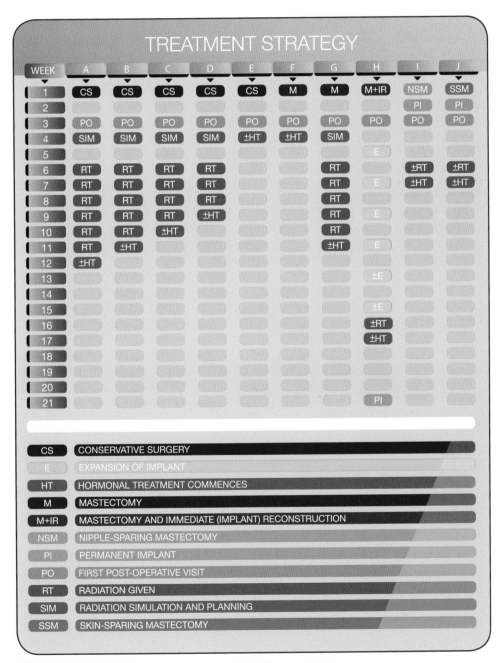

Figure 16.1 Overall treatment strategies available for your DCIS.

This next visit, after your consultation, is for radiotherapy simulation. This can be quite scary. The doctors and the technicians go through this every day, and hopefully they are sensitive to your fears (Figure 16.2). Behind the scenes, "Radiation Planning" takes place to plan a course of radiation beams, doses, and directions for your body (Figure 16.3). In general, radiation therapy is given to the breast or chest wall using a **linear accelerator** (Figure 16.4); the lymph glands are not treated. It looks scary, but don't be afraid of it. It's just a man-made machine that you lie on; and you breathe in normally as treatment is given. It's an open machine in a large room, and it's not too claustrophobic.

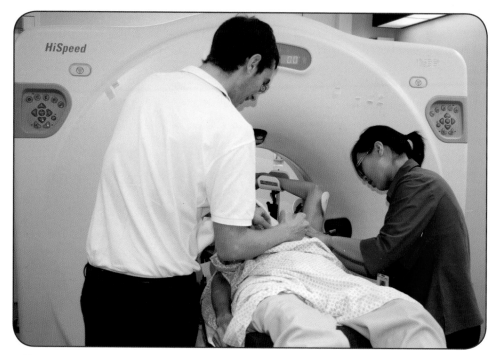

Figure 16.2 A CT scan is done during the radiation therapy planning procedure.

The machine is used by specially trained staff called **radiation therapists** or radiation technologists who position you carefully every day on the machine based on the prescription and plan approved by your radiation oncologist. The machine is operated using sophisticated computer controls. While the radiation beam is turned on, the radiation therapists can see and hear you through a closed-circuit television. The actual time it takes to give the radiation to each area is usually less than a minute, but each treatment slot may be ten to fifteen minutes long because of the time it takes to position you accurately using coordinates determined during the planning process.

How Much Radiation Is Given?

Radiation therapy is given daily (five days per week or sometimes five days one week and four days the next) for about four to six weeks. The standard dose of radiation given each day is 1.8 to 2.0 units. The amount of radiation absorbed by the tissues is called the **radiation dose** (called a Gray, or Gy). Some oncologists use the metric measure, called a rad. One Gy is equal to 100 **rads**. After

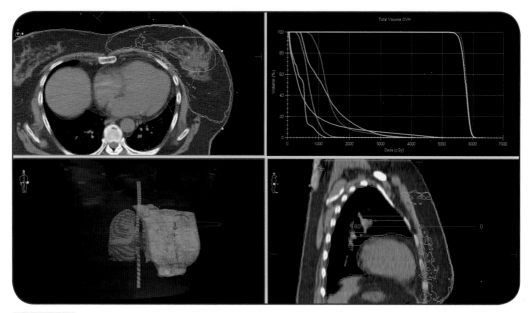

Figure 16.3 A radiation therapy plan is calculated specifically for your body using powerful 3D computer programs.

breast conservation, various dose prescriptions are used all around the world. A common dose used for the whole breast in the U.S. and Australia is 50 Gy over the course of 25 sessions ("**fractions**"). After 50 Gy, there is usually an extra week of radiation, at a dose of 2 Gy per day for five days. This is called a **boost**, and it's given to the **tumor bed** because this is where most recurrences in the breast tend to occur. A large clinical trial in Europe proved that women with invasive breast cancer who received a boost had a lower recurrence rate than those who did not. Given that what is left behind after a lumpectomy for invasive breast cancer is mainly DCIS, I suspect ongoing trials studying the value of a boost for patients with DCIS will show a small benefit.

Although no randomized trial has been published investigating the value of an additional boost dose for DCIS, a study from the Rare Cancer Network suggests the value of a boost in DCIS, especially for women aged under 45 years. Of the 373 women treated, 15% had no radiotherapy, 45% had whole-breast irradiation without a boost, and 40% had whole breast irradiation with a boost. With an average follow-up period of about six years, the 10-year recurrence rate in the breast was 53%, 28% and 14% respectively (Omlin 2006). Other studies have not found any benefit from a boost, but suggest that it be considered for younger patients or those with close margins (Wai et al. 2011).

Similarly, there are no published randomized trials of accelerated radiation following a lumpectomy for DCIS. However many oncologists are using higher doses of radiation given over three to four weeks rather than six to seven weeks based on the studies done for invasive breast cancer which show equivalent results (Whelan et al. 2010). A Canadian non-randomized study did not find that delivering 42.5 Gy in 16 fractions to be inferior to longer courses of radiation (Wai et al. 2011). To address these controversies, the Trans Tasman Radiation Oncology Group is conducting an international clinical trial randomizing patients to hypofractionated versus standard fractionated whole breast radiation, plus or minus a breast boost in patients with pure DCIS.

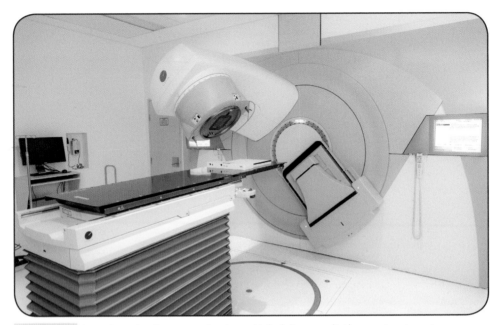

Figure 16.4 A modern-day linear accelerator, which delivers radiotherapy treatment.

Remember:

- You do not become radioactive from external-beam radiation.

- You can continue to hug and kiss your partner and your children.

- You will not glow in the dark!

- You are not more susceptible to infections.

- You can continue to work.

- You will not "beep" when you go through airport security.

- You need to attend somewhere between sixteen and thirty-three treatments.

The Radiation Therapy Planning Session

I usually let a patient's partner go in to the room to be with them for part of the procedure. At this planning session, which is also called a **simulation**, I always like to look at mammograms to see how big the area of DCIS was so that we can work out where to give the extra "boost" dose of radiation. Make sure you bring your X-rays along with you.

Most radiation therapy departments mark your skin with some permanent marks (tattoos) using a small amount of ink and a pinprick. The number of tattoos varies between departments. For example, where I work, we use four tiny tattoos. I avoid using the tattoo in the area of the neckline, which does make wearing low tops after radiation a little easier. Tattoos do fade with time and can be covered easily with cosmetic creams after treatment; or in rare circumstances, one that may be particularly bothersome to you can be surgically removed.

Many modern departments have what is called a CT simulator, and a planning **CT scan** is done right then and there. A CT is sometimes referred to as a "CAT scan" (Figure 16.2). The visit to the simulator will take about thirty minutes. You lie on a bed, and it takes X-ray "slices" of your body from around the middle of your neck to about 3 cm under your breast.

These slices are used to recreate a three-dimensional image of your upper body using a modern super-computer. The radiation doctor (often known as a radiation oncologist or radiotherapist) can mark where the cancer started (often marked by a titanium clip by your surgeon), where your breast is, and where vital organs such as the lung, heart, and spinal cord are located. Most of the planning work takes place behind the scenes over the next week using very complex mathematics done by a radiation therapist who specializes in computerized planning; such therapists are called **dosimetrists**, or radiation therapy planners in some countries.

Today we can restrict the amount of involved lung under your breast to small amounts. A small amount of involved lung is required to ensure that we don't undertreat the part of your breast that sits on your ribs just above your lung.

I think it is also important to minimize the amount of radiation that your heart gets. Sometimes it's simply not possible, but most times with modern three-dimensional radiation therapy, it's possible to protect all of the heart with special shields called **multileaf collimators**. Some departments also use special breath-holding techniques that push the heart backwards away from the chest wall behind the breast for left-sided cases, which are proving to be difficult. I sometimes use a type of three-dimensional arc therapy called VMAT (or Volumetric Modulated Arc Therapy) particularly for complex situations on the left side but this is rarely the case for DCIS (Figure 16.3). It's a bit like one of those smart sprinklers that can be programmed to change direction, water speed and pressure, and the number of outlets used depending on if it's facing the path or your garden. Similarly, VMAT-delivered radiation can sweep across and provide lots of shielding and reduce the dose rate when it's facing your heart and lung and then can also slow down and give increased doses when it's just treating your breast or chest wall. It does give more low-dose radiation to more of your body than conventional techniques. A video from the company that developed this technology is available from www.elekta.com/healthcare-professionals/products/elekta-oncology/treatment-techniques/delivery-techniques/elekta-vmat.html.

It's not always easy, though, so don't be too hard on your radiation oncologist. Some women have barrel chests and have more lung in the field than normal. Other women's hearts might be big because of early heart failure. Sometimes the location of the cancer makes it impossible to totally miss the heart, particularly when it's in the lower outer part of your left breast (i.e., the 4 to 5 o'clock position), or when it is located right next to the breastbone on the left side. It is really important to make sure that the area where the DCIS started is treated properly; and if that means some unavoidable radiation to the heart, don't be too worried—the risk of heart damage is still very low.

Common Side Effects during Radiation Therapy

Fatigue

You may feel tired during the treatment, particularly in the later weeks. Nobody really knows if it's just the radiation that causes this. A lot of my patients don't sleep all that well during this treatment because of the stress of the diagnosis and getting used to the fact that life has changed for the moment. Exercise may help with your fatigue.

Aches and Pains in the Breast

You may feel minor twinges in the breast for some time, often years. These are frequently sharp pains, usually in the scar. In my view, this is probably due to the nerves under the skin rejoining and causing some small electric shocks. There's not much you can do about this, apart from rubbing some vitamin E cream into your scar. Rest assured, though, that this should return to normal with time.

Swelling of the Breast

You may develop some fluid in the breast after your surgery and radiation treatment. This is called breast edema. Edema of the breast is particularly noticeable if you wear an underwire bra, which may cause an indentation of your skin. This is not dangerous. The areola area may become thickened with the edema too, and may feel more leathery and become paler, particularly in the first year or two. Breast lymphedema is not dangerous unless your breast gets infected and appears red and hot. If this occurs, see your doctor for some antibiotics.

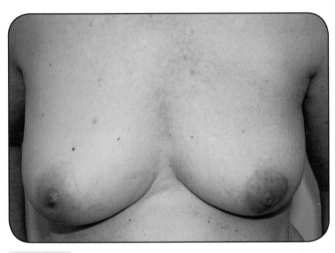

Figure 16.5 Skin reddening after week four of radiation to the left breast.

Breast edema is particularly common for large-breasted women and is worse in the first year after treatment, but it slowly improves by the third year. As with lymphedema of the arm, it is helpful to keep the breast moisturized. Some lymphedema therapists can train you to massage the fluid in the breast toward the breast bone, and this sometimes reduces the swelling.

Skin Reddening and Irritation

There may be some skin reddening by the second, but more usually the third or fourth, week of treatment (Figure 16.5), which will become more obvious and more diffuse by week five or six (Figure 16.6). The reddening may become a little worse over the

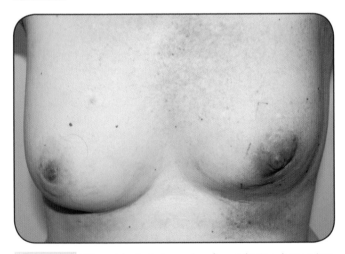

Figure 16.6 Skin reddening, six weeks after radiation, becoming worse over the scar ("boost" area).

area given the boost or extra dose in the week after the treatment finishes. This often occurs toward the breastbone and sometimes your outer nipple area as these areas receive a slightly higher dose of radiation therapy. After your course of therapy, it's not unusual for your breast skin to become slightly darker (particularly for people with darker skin). In the longer term, prominent blood vessels may appear in areas of skin that received a higher dose, and this is called **telangiectasia** (Figure 16.7). It is not dangerous. I recommend rubbing some bland barrier cream, such as vitamin E or even aloe vera, onto the skin on a daily basis.

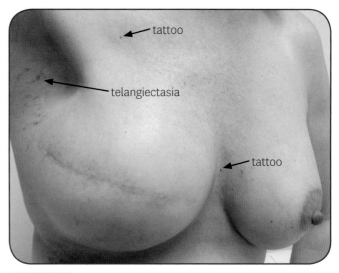

Figure 16.7 Prominent red marks, called "telangiectasia," over the skin towards the right armpit five years after treatment of the chest wall with an underlying implant.

Uncommon Side Effects during Radiation Therapy

Skin Reactions

Toward the end of the treatment, you may experience some blisters on your skin. These usually occur only in areas that have received a slightly higher dose. Because the breast is not a square block, the doses do vary across various parts of the breast. When you look at the radiation therapy plan, it's like a weather map with high- and low-dose areas. These days we tend to use what's called a "field-in-field", VMAT or IMRT (intensity modulated radiotherapy) technique where we use conventional fields to deliver most of the dose but then shrink the fields to come off areas where the dose is "hotter" which results in a more uniform dose. We look at all your breast in 3D views to ensure good dose uniformity. In the 1980s, we only looked at the center of your breast (called the "central axis") and tended to ignore the other areas because we did not have the supercomputers of today.

Parts of the breast which are not as wide as others (for example towards the nipple area) receive a slightly higher dose than other areas such as the back of your breast. Other areas that can get irritated more than others are those where skin folds rub against each other, such as under your breast or in the skin close to your armpit.

Modern radiation normally spares the skin, and the highest dose is about 10 mm under the skin. In some situations when we need to enhance the dose to the skin with tissue equivalent material (called bolus), the maximum dose is on the skin. This is done deliberately if we are worried about the cancer coming back on the chest wall after a mastectomy. The skin can get quite red in this situation, like bad sunburn, but it always settles down in two to four weeks.

Nausea

Nausea is quite uncommon. Radiation nausea tends to occur two to four hours after your treatment. You may feel queasy but rarely sick with radiation delivered just to the breast or chest area. If you are receiving radiation therapy to multiple areas, or if you're unlucky enough to have breast cancer in both your breasts, then this extra dose of radiation can cause radiation nausea.

If radiation nausea occurs, see your doctor about taking an antiemetic (antinausea) pill half an hour before your radiation treatment. Nausea and vomiting are more of a problem with chemotherapy than with radiation therapy. Drugs used to prevent nausea and vomiting include Stemetil (prochlorperazine), Maxeran (metocloparmide), or Cesamet (nabilone).

If you are receiving radiation therapy to other parts of your body and experience more severe nausea, then agents such as Zofran (ondansetron) can control it.

Rib Problems

Rib fractures are very rare, but very occasionally a woman may get a fracture in the treated area. More often than not, it's just tenderness over the ribs. I find that a lot of women develop what is known as costochondritis, common symptoms of which include sudden, severe pain and soreness, usually around the breastbone. The pain of costochondritis increases when pressure is applied to the tender area where the cartilage connects the ribs; it also increases with coughing, sneezing, or deep breathing, all of which move the cartilage or the ribs.

If a rib fracture does occur, it can be diagnosed by a **bone scan**, an X-ray, or both. Rib fractures usually happen twelve to forty-eight months after radiation therapy. On a nuclear bone scan, the ribs may show up as an abnormal "hot spot" indicating increased bone activity, often in a straight line in the region between the edge of your breast and your armpit. The important thing to remember is that it's very rare to get bone cancer that's spread from the breast in an area that's already had radiation therapy.

Some doctors may believe that the "hot spot" is cancer as they may not know that you've had radiation therapy to the area. If in doubt, a CT scan with "bone windows" or "bone settings" may clarify the situation.

Rib fractures nearly always heal and are not a serious complication. Both costochondritis and rib fracture can be helped with rest, warm compresses, and the use of anti-inflammatory medications (such as aspirin, ibuprofen, naproxen, or ketoprofen).

Lung Inflammation

In order to treat the breast, a small amount of lung needs to be treated so that we don't underdose the back of your breast. The whole breast needs to be treated, either by removing it or by giving all of it radiation therapy.

Radiation "pneumonitis" is rare. About one woman in every 200 may develop lung inflammation, usually six weeks to six months after therapy for DCIS. Symptoms include coughing and shortness of breath. A telltale sign is that you may feel excessively tired.

Long-term scarring can occur, but only in a very small area of the lung. All doctors treat this a little differently, and one size doesn't fit all. This is what I do:

- Perform a chest X-ray (and sometimes a CT scan) to confirm that nothing else is going on.

- Start some antibiotics, usually just simple Augmentin (amoxicillin, 500 mg, four times a day).

- Commence prednisone at a dose of 20 mg a day and reduce the dose by half every three days.

Other Cancers

Women who have had radiation therapy may be susceptible to other cancers. There is a slightly increased risk of ovarian cancer, for example, if there is a family history of breast cancer, which may indicate genetic susceptibility to breast and ovarian cancer. This is not due to the radiation therapy.

Sometimes, body fat breaks down around the scar, and when the fat dies and liquefies, this is called "fat necrosis." The body can calcify this area, and sometimes it may look like a recurrence, but it is nothing to worry about.

Very rarely, radiation may cause cancer. This is known as a **sarcoma** and can even occur after a mastectomy. Estimates vary, but one report suggests that there is one case in every five to ten thousand women, usually five to ten years after treatment (Marchal et al. 1999). But remember, this is like getting struck by lightning. I have seen three cases in thirty years. Assume it won't be you.

It's important to do a biopsy of any new tumors in the breast, particularly when they occur in the second five years, to exclude this more serious type of cancer. A recent report suggested a slightly higher risk of lung cancer if you have radiation for breast cancer. More research is needed, but if you smoke, try to stop or at least cut back.

Excessive Shrinkage of the Breast

About one in one thousand women may be more sensitive to radiation, and the breast may shrink quite substantially. There is really no way to know if this will happen. It tends to be more of a problem with larger-breasted women. If this occurs, plastic surgery may be able to help. Very rarely, a mastectomy will need to be done in this situation. The more common situation is shown in Figure 16.8. This is a photograph taken seven years after radiation. There is a slight amount of persistent pigmentation over the

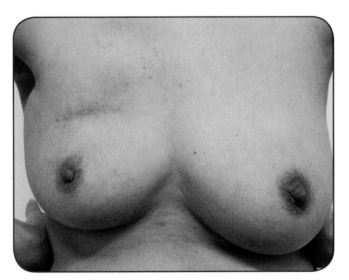

Figure 16.8 Shrinkage of the breast and increased skin pigmentation can occur after radiation.

scar, and shrinkage of the treated right breast made worse by gaining weight and depositing fat in the untreated breast but not the treated breast.

Pain in the Breast

Often, there are sharp or shooting pains, usually over the scar. They don't last long but may give you a bit of a scare. Sometimes a supporting bra helps these. Rubbing vitamin E cream into the scar may help in the longer term. These pains may occur in as many as seven out of ten women.

Breast-Feeding

After breast conservation, breast-feeding is usually not possible on the side where radiation was given, although a small amount of fluid may discharge from the nipple. Usually, the treated side stays smaller and the untreated side becomes larger and droops more. Otherwise, there is no problem with breast-feeding, provided you are not having chemotherapy.

Tenderness over the Pectoralis Major Muscle

Sometimes women get pain over the pectoralis (pec) muscles. The pec can be found by holding the muscle at the front of your armpit. These pains are not uncommon and are usually caused by some scarring of the muscle from radiation therapy. Because the pectoralis muscle is close to the surface, it does receive a slightly higher dose, and this can sometimes cause some discomfort and lack of mobility. Massage of the area by a physical therapist may help, as may rubbing vitamin E cream into the area regularly and continuing your shoulder exercises.

Skin Care during and after Your Radiation Therapy

This will vary according to your local treatment team. What you can do for yourself includes the following:

- Use a very mild soap, such as baby soap, Dove®, Ivory®, Cetaphil®, Neutrogena®, Basis®, Castille®, Aveeno® Oatmeal Soap or other similar soaps.

- Use warm water when you shower or bathe instead of very hot water.

- After showering, pat the skin dry rather than rub.

- Simple barrier creams such as Sorbolene (Australia, U.K.), vitamin E cream, Aqueous cream or Eucerin are helpful. Do not use creams that contain excessive cosmetics or perfumes. Some of my patients use calendula (Pommier, 2004). Rub your preferred cream into your treated area every day after treatment and before you go to bed. If your radiation treatment is in the afternoon, you can use your cream in the morning. Basically, the technicians who treat you need your skin to be dry when they treat you as they sometimes have to use marker pens to set you up every day.

At the beginning of treatment, before you have any side effects, moisturize the skin after your daily treatment with an ointment such as A&D, Eucerin, Aquaphor, Biafine, or RadiaCare. You also can put it on at night—wear an old T-shirt so the ointment doesn't get on your bedclothes.

Here are a few more tips:

- For mild pinkness, itching, and burning, apply an aloe vera preparation. Or try 0.5% to 1% hydrocortisone cream (usually available without a prescription at any drugstore). Spread the cream thinly over the affected area three times a day. Some of my patients use natural plant aloe vera, which is also helpful but a little messy.

- If areas become red, itchy, sore, and start to burn, and low-potency cream no longer relieves your symptoms, ask your doctor for a stronger steroid cream available by prescription. Examples include 2.5% hydrocortisone cream or betamethasone.

- Some women get some relief by blowing air on the area with a hair dryer set to "cool" or "air." Don't turn it to "heat."

- Don't wear a bra if there are raw areas, unless you cover them with some burn cream and a pad. If your skin forms a blister or peels in a wet way, leave the top of the blister alone! The bubble keeps the area clean while the new skin grows back underneath. If the blister opens, the exposed raw area can be painful and weepy. Keep the area relatively dry and wash it with warm water only. Blot the area dry and then apply a non-adherent dressing, such as Xeroform dressings or "second skin" dressings. To relieve discomfort from blistering or peeling, take an over-the-counter pain reliever, or ask your doctor for a prescription if you need one.

- I normally do not recommend aluminum-based deodorants during radiation therapy. There are some natural deodorants around, including tea tree oil and an ingredient called rock salt. Again, this is probably just a myth, but theoretically, the aluminum in the deodorants may interact with the radiation therapy and cause a more severe skin reaction. However, if it's the middle of summer and the natural deodorants are not working, perhaps a spray deodorant may be the best approach. Prantal Powder may also be used instead of deodorant.

- Do not shave under the arm with a razor blade on the treated side. You can use an electric shaver. The problem with shaving is that it can introduce infection with very superficial skin cuts.

- If radiation therapy is given to the armpit area, the sweat glands can become dry and some patients stop sweating on that side. Sometimes the hair doesn't grow back. Many women think this is a bonus! Apply a barrier cream to the areas of dry skin.

- Speak to your breast care nurse about the best bra to use. There are bra specialists that can help you. Cotton bras are probably better than nylon bras, as the nylon can irritate the nipple area (Figure 6.5 on page 85). Sometimes just putting a large cotton handkerchief between the bra and your breasts will help. Many find wearing a bra towards the end of treatment is too abrasive and causes too much rubbing over sensitive skin.

- Cotton T-shirts or singlets are helpful. Some women prefer not to wear a bra, particularly if small-breasted. If you're large-breasted, good support is necessary, and sometimes a sports bra is helpful.

- For large-breasted women, sometimes the fold between your breast and your abdomen (where the bra underwire normally goes) rubs just from the normal bounce of the breast, and this can be an area of irritation from friction. Putting a pad (such as sanitary pad or a Telfa pad) between your bra and your skin may help to protect this area, as may applying some Paw Paw gel (derived from the papaya tree, if available in your country), aloe vera, or creams such as Eucerin, Lubriderm, or Aquaphor.

- If you're having treatment in the area above the collarbone, the radiation can "exit" through your upper back and that area can become itchy. Make sure you rub Sorbolene cream into the area above your collarbone and also around the top of your back.

- If the skin peels, there are special creams used by the radiation therapy department. They do vary, but they include superficial burn creams (SSD cream, Solugel, or Paw Paw). Some of these creams need a dressing on top as they are quite sticky, but they are soothing.

- Don't expose your treated skin to extreme temperatures, including hot water bottles, electric blankets, or ice packs.

- A short swim in salt water is usually no problem during radiation therapy, but chlorinated water may irritate the skin. If you do take a swim in your pool, keep it short and pad yourself dry with a soft towel. Having said that, one of my patients insisted on swimming three kilometers a day during her radiation and her skin reaction was no worse than normal.

- After treatment, continue to moisturize the skin of your breast, chest wall, and arm at least once a day if possible.

- You will need to use sun protection cream or wear a sun protection T-shirt. Minimize sun exposure in the middle of the day and make sure you wear protective clothing, sunglasses, and a broad-brimmed hat.

- However, it's important not to wrap yourself up in cotton wool; try to get back to normal as quickly as possible.

As mentioned, much of this advice does vary from center to center, and it's important to talk to your own treatment team about their specific recommendations. Although it may be daunting at first, radiation treatment is usually over fairly quickly. One of my patients once explained that radiation is like a six-week vacation: before you know it, it's over and you're back at work.

CONTROL POINT #16 – DO I NEED RADIATION THERAPY?

WARNING

Treatment of your DCIS with a lumpectomy and without radiation increases your chances of DCIS or invasive breast cancer coming back in the breast. Always make sure you seek the opinion of a radiation oncologist as well as a surgeon.

TIP

You may feel minor twinges in the breast for some time, often for years, particularly around your scar. They are not a sign that the cancer has come back.

REMEMBER

Radiation therapy after breast conservation has been proven to be very effective provided that clear margins are achieved after your surgery.

Daphne's Story

When reflecting on my treatment of DCIS, the most outstanding memories are of the personal aspects of the treatment. I consider myself lucky to have been referred to my multidisciplinary team. I was particularly impressed with being introduced individually to each team member as they described their own roles. However, what I remember most of that day, and this still brings tears to my eyes when I remember it, was one young nurse at the foot of the bed whose role had not been described. I asked her, "What are you here for?" She replied, "I am here to hold your hand." And she did.

I found that the most important and reassuring elements of the treatment were the efforts of the medical professionals to explain simply and clearly each step of the treatment. So from day one I knew about the surgery and also how many radiation treatments I would have. For me, it was important to get a clear picture of what to expect. However, I believe we all face such issues in our own way and there is no "right" approach—only the one that is "right" for us.

Again the radiation therapy was made far less frightening and stressful by the unfailing kindness and respectful attitude of the staff at the hospital. I don't think that enough attention is given to the therapeutic benefits of having caring and supportive medical and allied health staff.

I was fortunate in being able to choose my time for daily treatment. If this is possible within the radiotherapy department, it is a great help to the patients. Because I had to travel quite a distance on a very busy freeway, I chose a very early appointment so the trip was less stressful. It also meant that it was so early that the radiotherapy team was running on schedule and parking was readily available.

My partner took me most days but once a week a friend went with me. Afterwards, we rewarded ourselves with a shopping trip and then we all had a special coffee treat. I know I could have driven myself, but it was comforting to accept the care of others. I did become too tired to go to the gym after a few weeks, so I took up a gentle exercise, tai chi, and have enjoyed it ever since.

I know it sounds like a cliché to say "Be kind to yourself," but I think it is a good principle during stressful times like this. Also, be ready to accept help from family and friends as, sometimes, it is a kindness to them as well as to yourself to allow them to help.

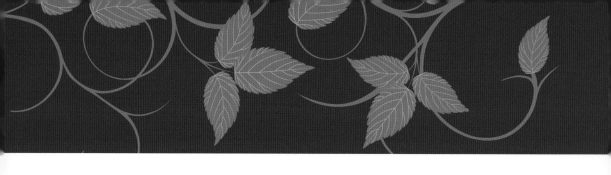

CONTROL POINT #17

DO I NEED HORMONAL TREATMENT?

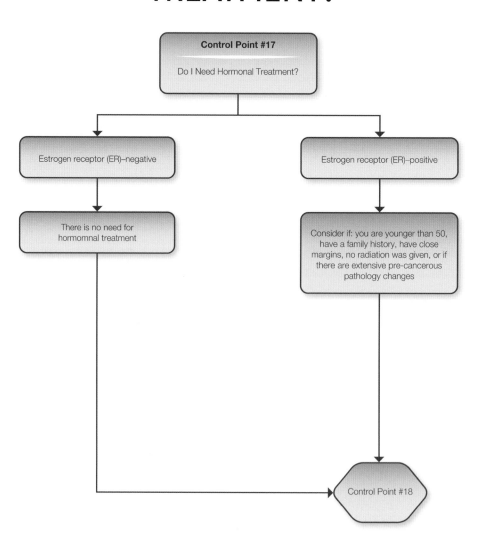

Control Point #17

Do I Need Hormonal Treatment?

Estrogen receptor (ER)–negative

Estrogen receptor (ER)–positive

There is no need for hormomnal treatment

Consider if: you are younger than 50, have a family history, have close margins, no radiation was given, or if there are extensive pre-cancerous pathology changes

Control Point #18

Do I Need Hormonal Treatment?

For the past thirty years or so, we have used antiestrogen treatments to try to prevent breast cancer spreading to other parts of the body. One aspect we discovered for patients with invasive breast cancer was that tamoxifen reduced the chance of breast cancer coming back in the same breast after radiation, in the chest wall after a mastectomy, and in the opposite breast.

It was logical, therefore, to extend this research to women with DCIS. What is clear to me is that most women with DCIS probably don't need tamoxifen. I will also briefly touch on the evidence that drugs like aromatase inhibitors, which stop the production of the small amount of estrogen produced by postmenopausal women, may also be helpful in the future. However, if you have an ER-positive DCIS or have other risk factors for developing breast cancer in the future, like a family history or perhaps an inherited fault in the breast cancer gene BRCA2, I think it's a good idea to think about whether tamoxifen may be worthwhile in your situation.

In this chapter, I will explain how estrogen that is produced in your body, even after you go through menopause, can act as a "fertilizer" and feed ER-positive breast cancer cells or their precursors (including DCIS or hyperplasia) that may be present in one or both of your breasts. Reducing the level of estrogen or blocking it from working can help stop these cells before they become a problem.

How Estrogen Is Made in the Body

Estrogen is a hormone produced by the ovaries until you reach menopause, and produced in small quantities by the adrenal glands, fat, and muscle tissue before and after you've gone through menopause.

You can see how estrogen is produced in Figures 17.1 and 17.2 below, which show some of the hormones produced by the different glands in your body. Basically, in the brain, an area just above the pituitary gland called the hypothalamus stimulates the pituitary with a compound called "luteinizing hormone releasing hormone" (LHRH), which then produces pituitary hormones called "follicle-stimulating hormone" (FSH) and "luteinizing hormone" (LH). FSH and LH stimulate the ovaries and the pituitary hormone "ACTH," which then stimulates the adrenal glands. In short, these hormones stimulate the ovaries to produce "female-type" hormones called estrogen and progesterone, and also the adrenal gland (mainly an issue in women who have gone through the menopause) to convert a "male-type" hormone called androgen to estrogen in very small amounts using an enzyme called aromatase.

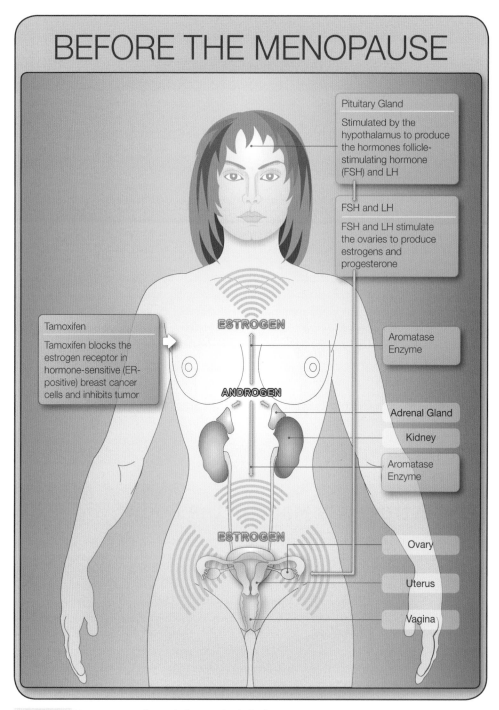

BEFORE THE MENOPAUSE

Pituitary Gland

Stimulated by the hypothalamus to produce the hormones follicle-stimulating hormone (FSH) and LH

FSH and LH

FSH and LH stimulate the ovaries to produce estrogens and progesterone

ESTROGEN

Tamoxifen

Tamoxifen blocks the estrogen receptor in hormone-sensitive (ER-positive) breast cancer cells and inhibits tumor

Aromatase Enzyme

ANDROGEN

Adrenal Gland

Kidney

Aromatase Enzyme

ESTROGEN

Ovary

Uterus

Vagina

Figure 17.1 How estrogen is made in your body before menopause.

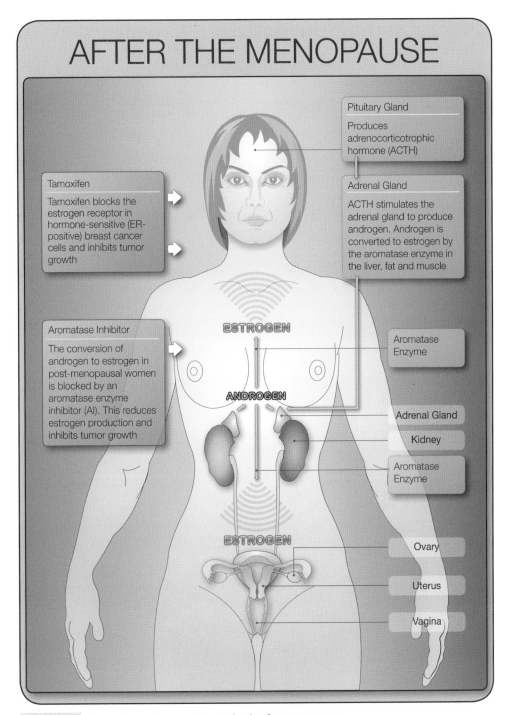

Figure 17.2 How estrogen is made in your body after menopause.

Understanding the Estrogen Receptor

There are a few different ways in which we can block the effect of estrogen or lower estrogen levels. Even though we call the treatment "hormonal therapy" or "hormone therapy," we really mean "anti-hormone" therapy because what we are trying to do is to reduce the level of estrogen in your body to stop it from stimulating the estrogen receptor. That's why I call it "hormonal treatment," so it's not confused with "HRT" or hormone replacement therapy, which is when extra estrogen is taken after the menopause.

I sometimes compare this estrogen pathway to how a television works. The very large broadcast antenna at a television network (e.g., BBC in the U.K. or ABC in the U.S.) is like your pituitary gland, which controls two smaller repeater antennas (the ovary and the adrenal gland) that send out the signal to your home.

The aerial antenna on the roof of your house is like the estrogen receptor, and the television in your living area is like the cancer cell. Houses with antennas are a bit like ER-positive breast cancer. If they get the signal, the television works when you press the "power" switch. Similarly, ER-positive breast cancer can be turned on by the estrogen that is normally made by your body. An ER-negative breast cancer is like the houses getting cable television with no antenna (Figure 17.3).

The aim of hormonal treatment is to "starve" breast cancer or DCIS cells of the hormone (estrogen) that may stimulate them to grow. Long-term research has shown that stopping estrogen from

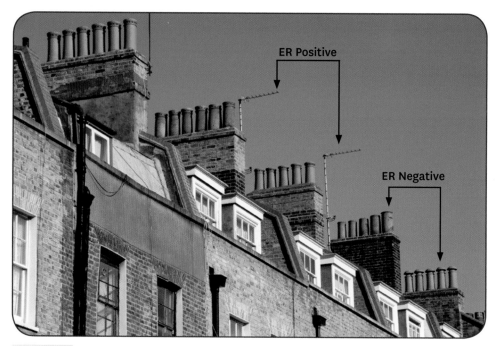

Figure 17.3 The television antenna system is a bit like the estrogen pathway in your body—stopping estrogen from reaching an ER-positive DCIS cell is like putting a lead shield around your roof antenna stopping your television from working.

stimulating any leftover hormone-sensitive cells lowers the risk of cancer coming back in the breast treated for DCIS as well as the other breast.

The only tested approach for women before they reach the menopause has been the use of the antiestrogen tamoxifen. Antiestrogen medicines do not decrease estrogen levels. Instead, they prevent estrogen from causing the DCIS cells to grow by blocking the estrogen receptor that may be present within the cell. These work a bit like putting a lead shield around the aerial antenna on your roof. The signal from the main transmission antenna is still there, but it can't make contact with your television antenna, so your television stops working.

Drugs or treatments that lower estrogen levels in the body include the **aromatase inhibitors** (such as anastrozole [Arimidex], letrozole [Femara], or exemestane [Aromasin]). Removing or stopping the ovaries from working is like knocking out one of the repeater antennas receiving the television network broadcast signal, which stops your television from working. These drugs are still being tested for women with DCIS but are likely to also work (Morrow 2012).

Antiestrogen Drugs: Tamoxifen

Tamoxifen has been used for over thirty years and is a true and tested drug in the treatment of breast cancer. Tamoxifen is also known as a **selective estrogen receptor modulator (SERM)** because it acts like estrogen on some tissues but blocks the effect of estrogen on other tissues. Tamoxifen (Nolvadex) and raloxifene (Evista) are two examples of SERMs. Both of these drugs have been used in trials involving women with a strong family history of breast cancer and have shown less DCIS and invasive breast cancer appearing. Given that they do work in a preventative setting, it makes sense to look at these drugs for women with DCIS.

Estrogen (shown in orange in Figure 17.4) is used by the cell if it finds a receptor inside the cell in its nucleus or nerve center. The estrogen receptor complex activates the cancer cells' genetic code or "DNA" of any cancer and can cause it to grow. Tamoxifen (shown in red in Figure 17.4) blocks the receptors in breast tissue and stops estrogen from working. Basically, tamoxifen works by "pretending" it is estrogen and binding to the estrogen receptor. Because it is a weak estrogen, it can sometimes stimulate estrogen receptors in other parts of the body, such as your womb, and in very rare circumstances cause unwanted side effects such as polyps or even cancer of the womb.

How Is Tamoxifen Taken and for How Long?

Tamoxifen is taken by mouth. The usual dose is 20 mg a day, and it's usually started after surgery or after the completion of radiation treatment. You can take tamoxifen with or without food, at any time during the day, but you should take it at the same time each day. If you like to take tablets in the morning ("to get them out of the way for the day") just add them to any other medications you may be taking. If you prefer to take tamoxifen at bedtime, that's fine as well.

You should not become pregnant or breast-feed while taking tamoxifen, or for two to three months after stopping. While tamoxifen can sometimes stop your periods and you may feel as if you've gone through menopause, you may indeed still be fertile. You should use some form of contraception other than the oral contraceptive pill, like a barrier contraceptive (condom or diaphragm), because the pill may alter the effects of the tamoxifen (see "Control Point #18 – Life after DCIS").

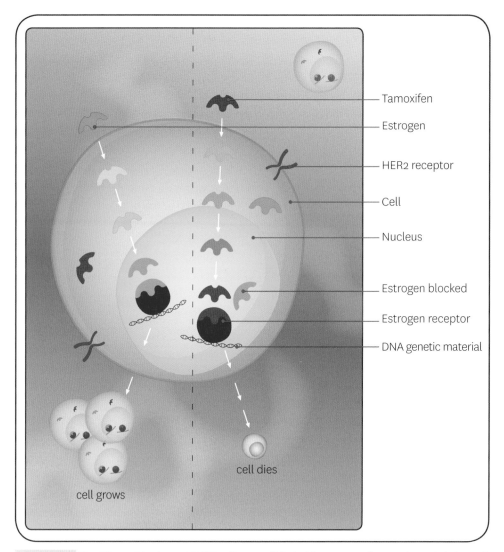

Tamoxifen

Estrogen

HER2 receptor

Cell

Nucleus

Estrogen blocked

Estrogen receptor

DNA genetic material

cell dies

cell grows

Figure 17.4 The ER-positive breast DCIS cell grows if fed with estrogen (orange), or shrinks and dies from estrogen being blocked by tamoxifen (red).

Currently, the recommended length for tamoxifen therapy is five years (Davies et al. 2013). A recent study suggested ten years may be better for patients with invasive cancer, but there have been no studies comparing different durations of treatment for women with DCIS.

What Are the Benefits of Tamoxifen?

Tamoxifen treatment can reduce the chance of breast cancer returning after breast surgery if you have DCIS that is ER-positive. It acts against the effects of estrogen in the breast, but as mentioned, it may act like estrogen in other tissues, so it may also provide some of the beneficial effects of estrogen. Some studies have found that it reduces the risk of heart disease by lowering cholesterol and may also reduce the chance of **osteoporosis.**

The benefits of tamoxifen are limited, and I will now present the available studies that have tested tamoxifen for women with DCIS.

Probably one of the best studies is one from the U.K. and Australasia as the investigators tested the benefit of tamoxifen with or without radiation after a wide local excision of DCIS.

The latest publication from January 2011 presented the results after an average follow-up of almost thirteen years.

Between May 1990, and August 1998, 1,694 women were randomly assigned to radiotherapy and tamoxifen, radiotherapy alone, tamoxifen alone, or to no adjuvant treatment (Cuzick 2011). The study examined the risk of either DCIS or invasive cancer coming back (which they called a "breast event") in the same or the opposite healthy breast. The risk of a breast event in the same breast after surgery alone was 26%, reduced to 20% if tamoxifen was added, 9% if radiation was added, or 6% if radiation and tamoxifen were added.

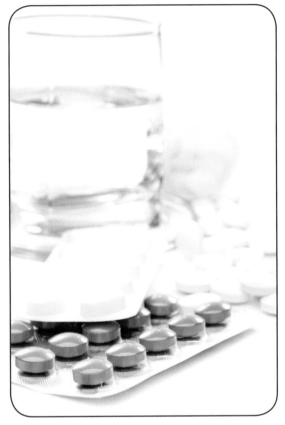

Taking a hormonal tablet means an extra tablet a day.

In terms of a more serious *invasive recurrence* in the same or opposite breast, the rates were as follows:

- No additional therapy: 14% (10% same side and 4% opposite side)
- Tamoxifen: 10% (9% same side and 1% opposite side)
- Radiotherapy: 6% (4% same side and 2% opposite side)
- Radiotherapy & tamoxifen: 5% (3% same side and 2% opposite side)

For recurrence of DCIS in the same or opposite breast, the rates were as follows:

- No additional therapy: 18% (16% same side and 2% opposite side)
- Tamoxifen: 12% (11% same side and 1% opposite side)
- Radiotherapy: 6% (5% same side and 1% opposite side)
- Radiotherapy & tamoxifen: 4% (3% same side and 1% opposite side)

So, you can use the numbers above to work out all breast events or you can flip it the other way and only look at the more serious events, which are the invasive recurrences. When you do that, you can see that the difference in invasive recurrence in this study was only 1% (6% for radiotherapy and 5% for radiotherapy and tamoxifen).

In my practice, I tend to use radiation almost routinely as I believe a risk of recurrence in the same breast of nearly 30% at thirteen years is too high unless you have a whole lot of other health problems. However, tamoxifen is not always easy and can cause side effects, particularly if you are aged between 40 and 55. If you have other risk factors such as younger age, close margins, a lot of other precancerous change (such as hyperplasia or lobular carcinoma in situ), or a first degree family history of breast cancer (i.e., involving your mother or father, sister, or daughter), then a trial of tamoxifen may be worthwhile. If you tolerate it, then keep it going for two years and continue to five years if you can. For women with invasive breast cancer, we know that five years of tamoxifen can reduce the future risk in the next twenty years. The decision is a little easier if your uterus has been removed as tamoxifen increases the risk of **endometrial cancer** a little. This is one of the main reasons (which I will discuss below) why scientists are testing aromatase inhibitors that do not increase the rate of endometrial cancer. We also know that the added benefit of five years of tamoxifen over two years is quite small.

The U.S. based NSABP group has examined the benefit of radiation with or without tamoxifen treatment in their B-24 trial (Wapnir et al. 2011). After 15-years, the recurrence rate in the affected breast was 18% for radiotherapy and only slightly lower with the addition of tamoxifen (16%). Once again, half of the recurrences were DCIS and half were invasive. Interestingly, in the other breast, recurrence was 11% for radiotherapy alone versus 7% with the addition of tamoxifen, suggesting a benefit with tamoxifen in reducing the risk of breast cancer or DCIS on the normal side.

Once again, it was found that tamoxifen in addition to radiation reduces the more serious type of recurrence by 1.5%, from 10% to 8.5%, fifteen years after initial treatment. This is not too different from the U.K./Australasia study which was 1%. Does that mean everyone should get tamoxifen? Probably not. The trial was also a little more complicated as one in four women had positive margins that we try to avoid today.

When the investigators just looked at the fifteen-year risk of an invasive recurrence by margins, the results were as follows:

- Positive Margins: Radiotherapy: 17.4%

     Radiotherapy & tamoxifen: 11.5%

So here is a situation where tamoxifen may help in addition to radiation. But, there was absolutely no benefit for women with clear margins, as shown below:

- Clear Margins: Radiotherapy: 7.4%

     Radiotherapy and tamoxifen: 7.5%

This trial showed that if your margins are clear, then the addition of radiation is all that is needed in reducing recurrence in the affected breast.

In another subgroup analysis, the authors found that most of the benefit from tamoxifen was for women under the age of 45 where the risk of an invasive recurrence with radiotherapy was 10% versus 3% when tamoxifen was also added. What we don't know, though, is how many of these younger women had a positive margin, which would have increased their risk. Furthermore, the estrogen receptor was not routinely measured, so I think this is probably a worst-case scenario.

On the one hand, we know there is more estrogen around when you are younger, and we also know, from Control Point #13, that eight of ten cases of DCIS are ER-positive; so, it sort of makes sense that tamoxifen may work better if you are younger. You also have more years at risk if you are younger and this may also increase the risk of getting a new DCIS or invasive breast cancer; or it may be that you may have developed DCIS earlier because you had a family history of breast cancer. On the other hand, tamoxifen can have side effects that are usually mild but can be wearing in younger women, such as hot flashes and night sweats, so a balancing act is required.

In summary, the NSABP trial suggests that the cost-benefit of using tamoxifen, in addition to radiation, may be worth it if you have close or positive margins, are under the age of about 45, and have other potential markers of future breast cancer such as a family history, precursor lesions in the breast (e.g., atypical hyperplasia), or lobular carcinoma in situ.

The last analysis of tamoxifen is a meta-analysis done by the Early Breast Cancer Trialists' Collaborative Group based in Oxford (Early Breast Cancer Trialists' Collaborative Group 2010). This group combined the data from the four randomized clinical studies that compared radiation to no radiation after surgery as discussed in "Control Point #14 – What Is My Prognosis?".

A total of 3,729 women were included in this meta-analysis, which combined all the studies and thereby probably increased the validity of the statistics. The risk of a recurrence in the breast was broken down at ten years after treatment with or without radiation or tamoxifen.

- No additional therapy: 29%
- Tamoxifen: 18%
- Radiotherapy: 13%
- Radiotherapy and tamoxifen: 9%

So, assuming a 50–50 split of invasive cancer versus a DCIS recurrence, the ten-year risk of an invasive recurrence with radiotherapy was 6.5% and with radiotherapy and tamoxifen about 4.5%, a difference of only 2%.

So, all the trials are basically pointing to a small benefit at most in reducing the risk of an invasive recurrence in the same or opposite breast by 1 to 2%. Thus, taking control at this point means questioning the use of tamoxifen in your own situation, or taking this book along and showing your doctor these trial results.

What Are the Side Effects of Tamoxifen?

Many women don't experience any side effects at all. The most common side effects are minor, and they usually lessen as treatment continues and cease when treatment stops.

Tamoxifen does not cause menopause, but its side effects are similar and can include:

- hot flashes (called "flushes" in the U.K., Australia, and elsewhere) or sweats
- irregular menstrual periods (if you have not gone through menopause)

- cessation of your menstruation

- vaginal irritation, dryness, or discharge

- fluid retention and weight gain. We don't really know if weight gain is due to the tamoxifen or just because people are getting older and may be less active. In one study where tamoxifen or a sugar tablet (placebo) was given to women who only had a family history of breast cancer to see if it could prevent breast cancer, both groups of women gained weight.

Uncommon side effects may include light-headedness, thinning hair, aches and pains in the joints, dizziness, headache, and fatigue. These usually get better after taking tamoxifen for a few weeks. Taking a half dose tamoxifen (10 mg per day) for about four weeks and then going up to the full dose may help your body get used to these side effects. An allergic type rash is very rare, as is nausea. Some women (e.g., who are in a choir or sing) may experience a slight deepening of their voice, as can occur naturally after menopause.

A rare complication (less than 1 in 100 chance at ten years) is the development of cancer of the uterus (womb), also known as endometrial or uterine cancer. The additional risk of cancer of the uterus is about 1 per 1,000 women per year taking tamoxifen. So if you take tamoxifen for five years, the additional risk is 5 in 1,000, or 1 in 200. In other words, the risk is real but very low.

Any abnormal vaginal bleeding should be reported to your doctor, who will decide whether further investigation is needed. Spotting can occur in women who have not gone through menopause. A routine gynecological check is advised before you start tamoxifen. There does not appear to be any benefit to having routine pelvic scans such as ultrasound (they are usually abnormal while on tamoxifen and serve no real purpose) for women who are taking tamoxifen. An annual pelvic check and Pap smear is a good idea when you are on tamoxifen and as part of your general health.

The risk of thrombosis (a blood clot) or embolism (a blood clot that travels) is the same as the risk of blood clots for women on the birth control pill or hormone replacement therapy. Report any sign of leg swelling or pain to your doctor. I normally recommend stopping tamoxifen for about one week before you travel if you're going to be immobile for long periods of time (such as long flights, car trips, or surgery) to try to prevent blood clots (such as with the "economy class syndrome") but not all doctors agree with this recommendation. If you have not reached the menopause, keep in mind you may get a withdrawal bleed after stopping your tamoxifen. In the NSABP-B24 study that I mentioned above, the risk of a thrombosis was 8 per 1000 for patients who just had radiation therapy compared to 18 per 1000 for those who had tamoxifen and radiation therapy for their DCIS (Fisher 1999). So the risk is real but very low. Some ways of reducing your chance of a thrombosis are documented well by the National Health Service in the United Kingdom, www.nhs.uk/Conditions/Deep-vein-thrombosis/Pages/Prevention.aspx.

Very rarely, tamoxifen can result in depression or mood swings. If this occurs, it may be worthwhile to switch you from tamoxifen to something else. Also, fine facial hair may become more prominent on tamoxifen. The risk of **cataract** may increase slightly for women taking tamoxifen, although this occurs normally as people age regardless. Other eye problems, such as corneal scarring or retinal changes, have been reported in a few patients. A rare form of inflammation of the back of the eye can be serious. Stop tamoxifen immediately and see an eye doctor as soon as possible if you are having visual disturbances.

I have seen two patients in the past twenty-five years or so whose platelets dropped. Platelets are the cells in the blood that stop you from bruising. If you get unexplained bruising, stop the medication and get an urgent **blood count**. I have also seen one patient with a drop in her white cells (the cells that fight infection), but not to dangerous levels. In all these patients, the blood counts returned to normal after they stopped the tamoxifen.

Can Tamoxifen Be Used with Other Medications?

Tamoxifen can interact with warfarin (a drug used to prevent blood clotting), and you should remind your doctor if you're taking it because your blood levels may need closer monitoring for a while. Do not take other hormone treatments if you're taking tamoxifen, but continue to take any other drugs that your doctor has prescribed. Avoid paroxetine (Paxil), sometimes used for symptoms of menopause, as it lowers the effective levels of tamoxifen.

Can Tamoxifen Increase My Chances of Surviving?

It is difficult to be sure of the answer to this question. If it does improve cure rates, it is likely due to stopping invasive cancer returning in the same breast or preventing it in the other side. The Oxford meta-analysis showed that death rates from breast cancer did not differ a lot whether or not a patient had radiotherapy after surgery; but they did not look at the incremental benefit, if any, from tamoxifen. In a study with one of my colleagues (as mentioned in "Control Point #14 – What Is My Prognosis?") presented at the American Society for Radiation Oncology in 2011, we showed that the ten-year risk of dying from breast cancer was lower for patients having both radiation therapy and tamoxifen (1.5%) than for patients having tamoxifen alone after their surgery (3.4%) or having surgery and radiation without tamoxifen for DCIS (3.1%) (Stuart et al. 2011). So, I guess the answer to this question is probably yes; but, ideally, this sort of analysis should be done by the Oxford group who have all the individual data to be totally sure as we used compilation of results based on published data.

Other Hormone Receptor Blocking Agents

Raloxifene (Evista) is another drug that has been shown to reduce the incidence of breast cancer and the chance of breast cancer developing in women with a family history; but, as yet, there are no studies proving that it works once you have DCIS. At this point in time, we are not recommending raloxifene for women with DCIS, even for the treatment of osteoporosis. It has been approved in the U.S. and Australia for women with a strong family history of breast cancer who have reached menopause in an effort to reduce their chance of getting breast cancer in the future. In the NSABP Study of Tamoxifen and Raloxifene (STAR), raloxifene was proven to be about three-quarters as effective as tamoxifen in reducing the risk of invasive breast cancer and DCIS, with less cancer of the womb, less thrombosis, and less cataracts. Longer follow-up is required to make firmer recommendations regarding its use for patients with DCIS (Vogel 2010). One paper has suggested that, despite raloxifene being less effective than tamoxifen, it had substantially less other complications, which made it an overall better option for women at higher risk of future breast cancer or DCIS (Freedman et al. 2011).

Drugs That Lower Estrogen Levels: Aromatase Inhibitors

Aromatase inhibitors (AIs) stop the small amounts of estrogen produced in your body after you have reached menopause. Three drugs in this class are available for treatment of breast cancer: anastrozole (Arimidex), letrozole (Femara), and exemestane (Aromasin). These drugs work by blocking an enzyme (**aromatase**) that makes estrogen in postmenopausal women by helping to convert it from androgen produced in places like the adrenal gland (see Figure 17.2). They cannot stop the ovaries of premenopausal women from making estrogen because there is too much estrogen floating around for them to work.

For this reason, they are only effective in postmenopausal women. The aromatase inhibitors have been compared with tamoxifen as adjuvant hormonal treatment in several clinical trials for invasive breast cancer. As yet, they have not been approved for use for patients with DCIS, although there is a lot of interest in their use for various reasons.

Firstly, there was an interesting lab study from Japan that showed that estrogen levels are raised in low-grade DCIS and in the step before DCIS (hyperplasia). Aromatase levels were also increased, which is the likely cause of the excess estrogen production in and around the DCIS. Blocking the aromatase enzyme could therefore help not only at the level of the adrenal gland (as shown in Figure 17.2) but also within the abnormal breast tissue itself (Sasano et al. 2010).

We also know that aromatase inhibitors can work for patients with DCIS by looking at the available studies that have used them for patients with invasive breast cancer or for patients at high risk of breast cancer. For example, in a large study from the National Cancer Institute of Cancer Clinical Trial Group (NCIC CTG) over 4,500 women with a higher than average risk of breast cancer, who had reached the menopause, were allocated to either the aromatase inhibitor exemestane group or placebo ("sugar tablet") group. About 10% of patients in the study were patients with DCIS who had a mastectomy. After an average follow-up of only thirty-five months, a 65% reduction in invasive breast cancer incidence was seen and the incidence of invasive breast cancer and DCIS was 53% lower in the exemestane group. Further lesions, thought to be the possible step before DCIS including lobular carcinoma in situ, atypical ductal hyperplasia, and atypical lobular hyperplasia, were less common for women taking exemestane (Goss et al. 2011).

The number of patients that were needed to be treated with five years of exemestane to prevent one patient developing invasive breast cancer was projected to be twenty-six. In this setting, despite some musculoskeletal toxicity, exemestane was well tolerated with discontinuation for side effects in 10% with placebo and 15% with exemestane. At this early stage, there were no differences between the groups in terms of bone thinning or fractures, heart or clotting problems, cardiovascular events, other cancers, or treatment-related deaths. However menopausal symptoms such as hot flashes, fatigue, sweating, insomnia, and arthralgia were frequent among all the women in the study but were predictably somewhat more common in those taking exemestane. Also of potential clinical importance, more women in the exemestane group self-reported that menopause-related and sexual symptoms had worsened. We also know from numerous other studies that taking out the ovaries, adding tamoxifen, or adding an aromatase inhibitor reduces opposite breast cancer (Goss et al. 2011).

To look at this issue further, a few small studies have found that giving an aromatase inhibitor for two weeks before surgery to remove an area of DCIS reduced its biological activity when they compared the preoperative core biopsy to the final pathology after it was surgically removed (Bundred et al. 2010).

Recently, one prominent researcher has argued that exemestane may be a good option for patients who have had a mastectomy on one side for DCIS to reduce the risk of invasive cancer on the other side, particularly for women in their 60s who still have a uterus (Chlebowski 2012).

Women taking aromatase inhibitors should have a bone density study which measures risk of osteoporosis or bone loss. As with other drugs, aromatase inhibitors may cause some side effects. Among the possible side effects are nausea or vomiting, stomach pain, muscle cramps, diarrhea or constipation, dizziness, a general feeling of illness (malaise), weakness and fatigue, hot flashes, loss of appetite, difficulty sleeping (insomnia), reduced sex drive, vaginal dryness, and joint pain.

So where to from here? All the evidence points to a small but real benefit, but more research is being done. The U.S. NSABP B-39 trial is comparing an aromatase inhibitor (anastrozole) to tamoxifen for ER-positive DCIS after a lumpectomy and radiation. This will help clarify the situation, particularly looking at side effects between the two agents. In the U.K./Australasia IBIS-II DCIS study, women who have undergone breast-conserving surgery and radiotherapy for DCIS are being allocated to anastrozole, tamoxifen, or placebo for five years. The IBIS-II DCIS data will certainly help with our future decision making but will take many more years before it is published.

In summary, your risk of dying from invasive breast cancer after a diagnosis of DCIS is VERY small. You can reduce your risk a little more by adding tamoxifen, or if you cannot tolerate tamoxifen and you and your doctor want to have some extra insurance, perhaps it's worth taking an aromatase inhibitor.

CONTROL POINT #17 – DO I NEED HORMONAL TREATMENT?

 WARNING
It's a good idea to stop your hormonal treatments about one week before flying long distances or if you are immobilized for a time after any future surgery as they may increase your chance of blood clots in your legs. You may get a withdrawal bleed if you have not reached the menopause.

TIP
If you have an ER-positive DCIS, hormonal treatments such as tamoxifen should be considered after your surgery and radiation therapy, particularly if you are younger, or there is doubt about your margins, or there is an increased risk of breast cancer on the other side.

 REMEMBER
Hormonal treatments for DCIS help a little but not a lot, and your doctor may look at many factors to help you decide if the risk of complications is worth the potential benefit.

Vicki's Story

I was 55 when I was diagnosed with a large area of low-grade DCIS. This was removed with clear margins, and I finished radiation. My oncologist then spoke to me about some of the benefits of tamoxifen. He was concerned about the surrounding breast. There was a lot of areas of "hyperplasia," "atypia," and "LCIS," which can occur in both breasts. My mother and auntie had breast cancer, and I really didn't want to have both my breasts off. I read all the studies about tamoxifen and DCIS and decided to give it a try as a type of preventative agent to calm down my breasts. My doctor said to me, "Take it for eight weeks first and let's see if you have any side effects; then we will aim for one year, then three years, and, if all is OK, we will try and make it to five years." I took the tamoxifen for five years in total without any side effects and must admit felt a little nervous stopping it.

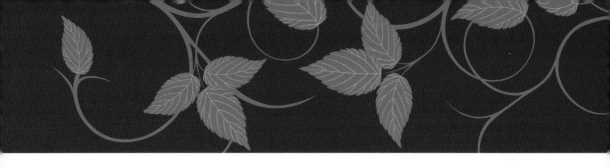

CONTROL POINT #18

LIFE AFTER DCIS

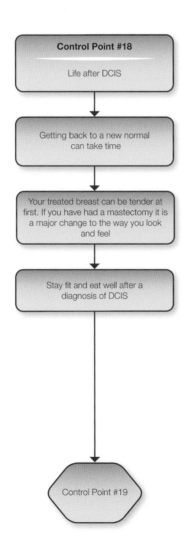

Control Point #18

Life after DCIS

Getting back to a new normal can take time

Your treated breast can be tender at first. If you have had a mastectomy it is a major change to the way you look and feel

Stay fit and eat well after a diagnosis of DCIS

Control Point #19

18

Coping with the Loss of Your Breast

There is no doubt that different women deal with this loss with different reactions. Breast surgery and radiotherapy can affect how women feel about themselves and their attractiveness. This can happen whether or not you have a partner. The changes to your body, how much energy you have, and your mood will affect how you feel about yourself. This includes your desire and ability to be sexual with others. You might feel less attractive because of breast surgery and radiotherapy. Or your breast might feel tender after treatment.

There are ways of dealing with these problems. Some suggestions are listed below.

- Try to talk with your partner about each other's fears and needs. This will help you adapt to your situation and feel closer to one another.

- Ask for advice, either together or separately, from a specialist, such as a relationship counselor, sex therapist, other counselor, psychologist, or psychiatrist.

- It's common to have sexual concerns after treatment for DCIS. If you or your partner has concerns, try to discuss these with your doctor, nurse, or other health care professional.

- If your doctor is unable to help you arrange a referral to a specialist, the Cancer Council Helpline (Australia) on 13 11 20 can provide information about specialists. In the UK, visit www.breast cancercare.org.uk or call their free helpline on 0808 800 6000 or call the Macmillan Support Line on 0808 808 00 00. In the U.S., the Cancer Information Service, www.cancer.gov or 1-800-4-CANCER, or the American Cancer Society, www.cancer.org or 1-800-227-2345, may point you in the right direction.

One study from Sweden looked at women's feelings toward their body image after conservative surgery (with or without radiation) compared to a mastectomy with an immediate breast reconstruction (Sackey 2010). Women treated for DCIS have a satisfactory long-term quality of life. The addition of radiotherapy to breast-conserving surgery did not seem to have any negative impact on quality of life. However, body image appeared to be affected for patients who had a mastectomy and an immediate reconstruction. Body image was studied using scores of ten items. For six items, women who had a mastectomy and immediate reconstruction felt more self-conscious, less physically attractive, less feminine, less sexually attractive, and more dissatisfied with their body and their scars than women who had breast conservation. For example, 73% of women who had a mastectomy and immediate reconstruction reported being self-conscious about their new body compared to 27% after conservative surgery and radiation. In terms of being sexually attractive, 73% who had a mastectomy and immediate reconstruction felt less sexually attractive compared to 31% who had conservative surgery and radiation and 21% who had breast conservation without radiation. It is likely, however, that reconstructive techniques that preserve the nipple (although no longer sensitive) may help improve these results. The authors concluded, however, that patients need more preoperative information about what changes in body image to expect after surgery.

Contraception after DCIS

Conventional wisdom is to stop "the pill" or other hormonal contraception after being diagnosed with DCIS, particularly if it is ER-positive. This may mean you need to use alternative contraception that may have implications for your relationship. Take care and continue to use barrier contraception (such as condoms or a diaphragm with spermicide) or intrauterine devices (IUDs). Some, but not all oncologists recommend an IUD that releases a small amount of a synthetic hormone into your womb every day.

I'd like to clarify two important points. Firstly, menopause is generally defined as the absence of menstruation for twelve months or more. But if you are on tamoxifen, it may be a "false menopause"; your periods can start again once you stop taking this medication. So just because your periods stop, particularly while on tamoxifen, do not assume that you no longer need contraception. Secondly, if your periods come back, it doesn't necessarily mean that you will still be fertile.

If you are taking tamoxifen, take extra care to avoid pregnancy. Tamoxifen can also stimulate ovulation, so don't rely on it as a contraceptive. In short, if you are taking tamoxifen and your periods stop, you may still be fertile, and you should use barrier-type contraception or an IUD. Furthermore, if you are under the age of 50 and your periods have stopped while on tamoxifen, it's best not to take one of the AIs (aromatase inhibitors; e.g., anastrozole, letrozole, or exemestane) mentioned earlier because they may, in fact, stimulate your ovaries to produce an egg (ovulation) and cause an unwanted pregnancy (Mourits et al. 2007; Smith et al. 2006).

Having a Baby after DCIS

A difficult and emotional issue to face is becoming pregnant after DCIS. Important issues for discussion include whether or not the pregnancy can cause harm from the associated increased estrogen levels. There have been a few case reports of problems, but most large studies have not shown an adverse effect on your prognosis from pregnancy after breast cancer. While many doctors advise waiting two years after treatment, there is no science to this whatsoever, and I have had many patients have children as early as six months after all treatment stops. It depends on factors such as your current age and the chances of your DCIS coming back. Even if your periods have returned, your chances of becoming pregnant may not be as high as they were before your breast cancer treatment. One important aspect to consider is that you may reach menopause earlier than you would have if you hadn't had DCIS after a course of tamoxifen.

If you are on tamoxifen, I suggest stopping it for at least two to three months before you try to get pregnant to ensure that it's totally out of your system. It's best to talk to your doctor about starting tamoxifen again after you have finished breast-feeding. If you have become pregnant while on tamoxifen, discuss this with your oncologist and obstetrician as soon as possible. The chance of damage to the baby is very low, but there have been only a few case reports of malformations (Berger 2008).

199

The hardest aspect of all this, though, is the awful thought of how you and your partner could look after yourself and a baby if by chance you had DCIS which then recurred as invasive cancer, or, in the worst case, you don't survive your DCIS or a subsequent invasive cancer. But remember over 97% of women with DCIS live a normal life. If you have good family support and feel that your partner could look after a child even if you were not around, then there is no reason to avoid the pleasure of having a child.

If you are considering having a child, you should be aware that:

- Breast-feeding will not be possible on the treated side.

- Your healthy breast will enlarge during pregnancy while the breast treated by lumpectomy and radiation will not change size or produce milk, which can result in an imbalance.

- The pregnancy will play a role in your follow-up tests. I normally organize a mammogram and ultrasound as it's impossible to see through the normal breast once you start breastfeeding. If you have any unusual symptoms elsewhere in your body, I normally recommend a CT scan and a bone scan just to be sure.

- The incidence of miscarriage or fetal abnormalities following treatment is not increased (Durrieu et al. 2004 & Kroman et al. 1997).

If you can't get pregnant, you may have to look at more difficult pathways, such as national or international adoption. Many agencies are not supportive of women with breast cancer adopting babies, but speak to your doctor about a letter of support. Most doctors are happy to do this given you have an almost normal life expectancy after DCIS.

Coping with Menopause

Menopause Symptoms after Breast Cancer Treatments

Symptoms of menopause are the most frequent and troublesome side effect after treatment of DCIS with hormonal treatment; or, you may be going through the menopause naturally after your treatment of DCIS by surgery with or without radiation therapy. Many women go through menopause without any problems at all, whereas others have a tough time with severe hot flashes and night sweats.

Usually your body can adjust to reduced estrogen, and many of these symptoms will improve on their own over time. It's hard at first when estrogen levels drop suddenly after treatment rather than gradually over time as they would with a natural menopause.

Common symptoms from reduced levels of estrogen in your body can be classified as follows:

Vasomotor

- Hot flashes and night sweats are common. They can be mild (occurring once or twice a day) or severe (more than twenty per day).

- Heart palpitations.

- Headaches.

Sexual

- Vaginal dryness and pain with intercourse are more typically problems with aromatase inhibitors, but they can occur after tamoxifen.

- Urinary frequency and occasional stress incontinence are not uncommon.

- Reduced sex drive is quite common, particularly during treatment.

Psychological

- Feeling down, tired, anxious, or irritable can be caused by menopause, particularly while you are feeling pressured during treatment.

- Poor sleep can be a direct side effect of hormonal treatments, particularly aromatase inhibitors, but is also secondary to menopause.

- Poor memory and concentration may be a direct menopausal effect or, more likely, may be related to sleep deprivation or a direct effect of hormonal treatments, based on a few small studies.

Somatic or Physical

- Bone thinning can occur from reduced estrogen. Consider taking calcium, vitamin D, or using a bisphosphonate if you have established bone thinning or loss. For example, taking zoledronic acid (Zometa) 4 mg intravenously every six months effectively inhibited bone loss for patients on aromatase inhibitors and even tamoxifen (Chien et al. 2006).

- Joint aches can occur and are best managed with stretching, exercise, and glucosamine. Sometimes antiarthritis tablets can help. In severe cases with an AI, it may be best to switch to tamoxifen or stop the drug altogether (Felson & Cummings 2005).

- Dry skin or a sensation of ants crawling under your skin ("formication") can also occur. This usually goes away on its own with time. Use a regular moisturizer even if it does get better.

Possible Treatments to Help Menopause Symptoms

1. Many things can aggravate hot flashes including stress, hot drinks, alcohol (particularly red wine), overheating the body in spas or baths, hot weather, and spicy foods. Both negative stress and positive stress (such as a party) can aggravate hot flashes. Avoiding these factors can help. Paced breathing with deep inhalations, holding for five seconds, and then breathing out slowly can help. This is a good way to relax. Find a quiet room and put on some calming music, and do this for about ten to fifteen minutes a day in one or two sessions. Relaxation techniques such as yoga or massage can help too. A Finnish study found that traditional Chinese acupuncture may be helpful (Borud et al. 2009). Wearing clothes made from natural fabrics such as cotton, silk, or linen in layers that you can take on or off as you get hot or cold is also practical.

2. Use of nonhormonal herbal therapies or vitamins such as Remifemin (an extract of Black Cohosh; two tablets morning and night), a red clover extract such as Promensil (one tablet a day), or vitamin E (800 international units [IU] per day) can sometimes help with mild hot flashes and night sweats. Always read the instructions and precautions before you take these over-the-counter drugs. Just because they are not prescription does not mean they cannot be dangerous if misused. Several

case reports of possible severe liver damage have been reported with Black Cohosh (making it unavailable in some countries), but millions of people use this every year so the risk is extremely low. Another alternative for mild symptoms is low dose clonidine (Catapres). The initial oral dose for hot flash treatment is 0.05 mg twice daily, but you may require at least 0.1 mg twice daily. The clonidine patch (delivering 0.1 mg/day) can also be considered, but it is not available in some countries. When discontinuing higher-dose therapy, gradually decrease the dose rather than stopping it suddenly. Clonidine has been used in higher doses for blood pressure control, but it can cause side effects, such as dry mouth, constipation, drowsiness, or difficulty sleeping.

3. If the hot flashes continue or are moderately severe, the same drugs used to treat anxiety and depression, such as venlafaxine (Effexor), can be helpful in lower doses. The starting dose is 37.5 mg daily for two weeks and then 75 mg daily. If it doesn't help within four weeks, it's best to try something else. I tend to start with this medicine if your symptoms are moderately severe (for example, more than ten hot flashes or episodes of night sweats a day), or if you have significant psychological effects or difficulty sleeping. Venlafaxine can cause weight loss by causing loss of appetite and may be preferred by overweight women for this reason. Reduced libido and difficulty achieving orgasm has been reported in about one in five women taking this drug for anxiety or depression (Kennedy et al. 2000).

4. Another drug in this class of medicines is paroxetine (Paxil), with a starting dose of 10 mg daily increasing to 20 mg daily after one to two weeks. It is best, however, not to take paroxetine if you are on tamoxifen, as paroxetine can make tamoxifen less effective by breaking down its active ingredient. Side effects, especially nausea and reduced libido, should be monitored. Reduced libido and difficulty achieving orgasm has been reported in about one in two women taking this drug for anxiety or depression (Kennedy et al. 2000).

5. A few case reports of increased libido have also been reported (Pae et al. 2005). Paroxetine is best taken at night because it sometimes causes drowsiness. Paroxetine has similar side effects to venlafaxine, although it causes less nausea and less loss of appetite. It can also rarely cause blurred vision.

6. Some doctors try other drugs such as gabapentin (Neurontin), which is used for nerve pain, up to 300 mg three times a day. I tend to start patients on a dose of 100 mg per day to be given at bedtime, particularly if you're over 65 as it can cause dizziness. If you continue to have hot flashes, the dose can be increased to 300 mg twice daily and then to three times daily, at two-week intervals. Antacids for heartburn can reduce the effectiveness of gabapentin, which should be taken at least two hours after antacid use.

7. If all else fails, some form of short-term hormone replacement therapy (HRT) may be needed. Progesterone tablets, such as low doses of Provera or Megace, are very effective in treating night sweats but are probably not safe to take for long periods because of their link to causing breast cancer when taken as a form of HRT with estrogen. However, a counterargument is that we used high doses of Provera as a form of treatment of breast cancer for many years in the 1980s. Certainly, if your tumor is ER-negative, it's probably safe as a short-term measure. If progesterone tablets fail, HRT such as tibolone (Livial), available in the U.K. and Australia, appears to be safe for women with ER-negative breast cancer, but a recent study has found that it increases the risk of cancer coming back if the original breast cancer was ER-positive (Kenemans et al. 2009). The problem with the study was that the number of patients in the study was small, so we can't be too sure of

the statistics just yet. In the U.S., low-dose estrogen therapy or estrogen and progestogen HRT may be considered in severe cases of menopause, but you need to be aware that this may increase the chance of your cancer coming back.

8. Vaginal estrogen can help with dryness and reduced vaginal tone, but it's probably best avoided if you're taking an aromatase inhibitor because, theoretically, the small amount of vaginal absorption may counteract the effect of the AI (Kendall et al. 2006).

Use water-based vaginal lubricants and moisturizers. Vaginal moisturizers such as vitamin E or Replens should be used on a regular basis after you shower to help hydrate and revitalize the vaginal lining and vulva. Krychman (2009) has advised that lubricants, especially those without flavors, colors, or warming additives, can and should be used during intercourse. He also notes that lubricants like Vaseline and oil-based products should be avoided since they can change the natural balance of vaginal bacteria and, in some women, may lead to infections. Excellent lubricants include Slippery Stuff and Sylk. Care should be used with Astroglide and KY Jelly, as some women find these products drying and the additives in them may be irritating.

The bottom line with all of this is to proceed with care. There is no right answer, and you need to balance your symptoms with the possible side effects and risks of taking some of these countermeasures. The evidence one way or the other is weak to say the least, so "taking control" here means understanding your options, talking to your treatment team, and seeing an understanding gynecologist for an examination and advice, preferably one who works with a breast cancer team.

Impact of Treatment on Sexuality

There hasn't been as much research into sexuality after a diagnosis of DCIS as there has been after invasive breast cancer, but many of the treatments are as aggressive and can, of course, have huge impacts on self-esteem and positive feelings about yourself after a diagnosis. There is no doubt that not going through the trauma of chemotherapy makes things a little easier, and there is no chance of an earlier menopause if you have not been prescribed tamoxifen.

A study from the Harvard School of Public Health specifically looked at 304 sexually active women who were treated with a variety of techniques after a diagnosis of DCIS. Sexual function in women with DCIS appears to be very similar to women in the general population and did not seem to be significantly disrupted by a diagnosis of DCIS. Sexual function and body image were notably stable across the eighteen-month length of follow-up. Women in this study who underwent mastectomy without reconstruction reported significantly higher average sexual satisfaction than patients who did not have mastectomy. Though this seemed paradoxical, the authors postulated that it was possible that women who opted to forego reconstruction may have been more comfortable with their bodies and had a greater sense of sexual satisfaction at baseline than their peers who did opt for reconstruction. However, the authors state that this was a small group of twenty patients and, therefore, more study is required in this group. Women who underwent mastectomy with reconstruction had the lowest sexual satisfaction scores immediately after their treatment; this improved slowly with time to reach identical levels of satisfaction as women who had breast conservation but still remained lower than the satisfaction levels of women who had a mastectomy. Importantly, tamoxifen use was not significantly related to lowered sexual function for women with DCIS (Bober 2013).

The diagnosis of breast cancer can affect the way you view yourself and your sexuality. Doctors often don't bring up sexuality because they may be concerned that doing so will extend the length of their consultation or because they may just feel uncomfortable talking about the subject.

Some health professionals equate sex only with intercourse, which of course is only one facet of human sexuality. Most of my patients do suffer at least a temporary reduction in sex drive and intimacy, and there is no doubt that this can put pressure on relationships. Often, there is an enormous loss of self-esteem following the loss of a breast, which is only partially helped by a reconstruction. A mastectomy can have different effects on different people. I've treated some patients who are comfortable lying topless on the beach after a mastectomy, whereas most feel a loss of self-esteem and become self-conscious about being seen nude. What I often observe is that women are more worried than their partner about losing their breast.

On the other hand, women who have breast conservation tend to feel more positive about their body image but may sometimes be left with an underlying sense of concern about cancer coming back in the breast that is left behind. Women who have breast conservation often do not appreciate their treated breast being caressed, particularly in the first year or two after treatment, because of increased tenderness and swelling. Nipple sensitivity can also be reduced temporarily or permanently after treatment.

Sometimes, there is a loss of libido (sex drive) that is temporary or has already been occurring for some time. If it persists, speak to your doctor or ask for a referral to an expert in this field. It's often hard to bring this topic up with your health professional, but you'll be glad you did. You can talk to a breast care nurse, if available, or try these questions or statements:

- I'm having problems with my relationship with my partner.

- I have vaginal dryness that is making sex less enjoyable.

- My sex drive has gone down, and I have lost interest in sex.

- What vaginal lubricants can I use?

- What are the symptoms associated with menopause?

- What should I do about contraception?

You have a right to information and nonjudgmental care. If you are not satisfied, ask for a second opinion from a relationship or sexual health expert.

I'm not a big fan of testosterone tablets or cream to try to increase sex drive as this can be converted to estrogen in the body and, theoretically, make matters worse. As mentioned above, sometimes drugs like venlafaxine (Efexor) or paroxetine (Paxil) that are used to help hot flashes can cause loss of orgasm. It's very important to work out the timing of your loss of orgasm with any new medications you may have been given.

Another factor that can affect sexuality is just feeling down, both during and after all your treatment. It is very normal to feel flat, sad, crushed, knocked down, sleep deprived, disorganized, or even that things are hopeless; but most people will just work these through and come out stronger and better equipped, usually without needing antidepressants along the way. Try to avoid antidepressants as a "quick fix" and instead seek to normalize your sleep patterns, become more active, organize "dates" with your partner, and schedule some regular activities such as going to the movies, meeting up with friends, or starting a regular walking group with your neighbors.

If you have problems getting to sleep, waking up early and not being able to go back to sleep, or just feel lousy and less motivated to do your normal routine, seek advice from your family doctor. Here are some ideas:

- Keep communicating about sex and intimacy.

- Use water-based vaginal lubricants during sex.

- Don't always have intercourse. External closeness, or "outercourse," is a good alternative, particularly as you start recovering from treatment.

- For partners, give your loved one a head-to-toe massage, which will help her relax and build up her self-esteem. It will be much appreciated.

- If you don't feel like sex, try to give your partner a massage and/or bring him or her to orgasm without intercourse.

- Take short breaks away, preferably without the children.

- Speak to your doctor about using vaginal estrogen if vaginal dryness is causing pain with intercourse.

- Exercise at least three times a week.

- If you have a sudden loss of sex drive and orgasm, check with your doctor about whether it could be treatment related.

- After treatment, look at buying some new, sexy lingerie and see a specialist bra fitter who is experienced with women who have had breast cancer.

- See a sex therapist if you are concerned about your situation.

- And, just to reiterate, keep talking to your partner; they will have their ups and downs too, and may feel lost and scared about the thought of losing you.

- Tell your partner that you will get through your treatment, and life will get back to some new normality where you can spend some time together deciding new priorities for yourselves, your relationship, and your lifestyle.

- Visit www.breastcancer.org/tips/intimacy.

- A good resource has also been developed by the Breast Cancer Network Australia (BCNA). Visit www.bcna.org.au/living-breast-cancer/sexual-wellbeing for more information.

Remember, your partner loves you because of you, not because of your breast. An important step is to show your partner the new you after your surgery. It's never easy at first. Most men do cope, but many can't communicate as well as you and need some prompting. Many relationships become strengthened after breast cancer; but sadly, a few fall apart.

If you are not in a relationship, finding a suitable and available companion is always a challenge—with or without DCIS or breast cancer. I've seen many, many success stories of women meeting new partners after breast cancer. Connecting and becoming friends is important in any relationship. When trust has been established, letting them know about your condition and what you have been through is very important. Be honest and put the issue "on the table." If they can't cope with it, you don't want to know them anyway and deserve much better.

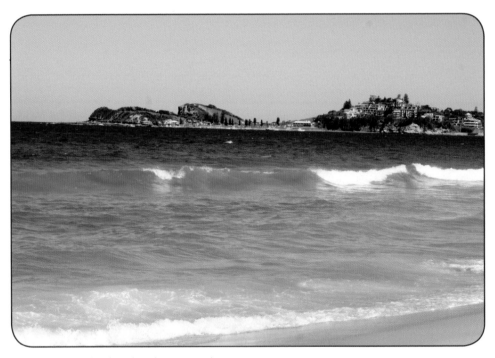

Remember to take short breaks away with your partner.

Staying Fit after a Diagnosis of DCIS

A report from Dana-Farber Cancer Institute in Boston examined exercise activity for 391 women at the point of their diagnosis of DCIS, and then again eighteen months later (Ligibel et al. 2009). Just before diagnosis, most women performed strenuous physical activity infrequently, and only half engaged in any type of exercise more than twice a week. Overall, activity patterns did not change greatly over the course of the study. Of note, women who underwent a mastectomy and those who were anxious at enrollment were far more likely to decrease exercise levels, and women who worked were significantly more likely to increase exercise over the course of the study.

Studies have demonstrated that many women gain weight after breast cancer diagnosis, putting them at higher risk of developing diabetes, heart disease, and other health problems. Data also suggest that overweight breast cancer survivors are more likely to develop additional breast cancers and other malignancies (Niraula 2012). Weight gain is most common in women treated with chemotherapy and in those who go through menopause as a result of cancer therapy; but studies also demonstrate weight gain in patients treated for DCIS and those who undergo surgery alone for early stage invasive cancers. It is not completely clear why women gain weight after breast cancer diagnosis, but several trials have suggested that reductions in physical activity may be at least in part to blame. Gentle exercise, like walking, is ideal, but some women find that more strenuous exercise is also helpful. Check with your doctor about the level of exercise that might be suitable for you.

Some good information is available from the Breast Cancer Network Australia Web site, www.bcna.org.au/living-breast-cancer/physical-wellbeing/exercise-staying-fit.

Getting Back to Work

If you worked or were involved in a regular activity when you were first diagnosed with DCIS, returning to this job or activity soon after treatment could make you feel valued and give you the comfort of being around people you're familiar with. You might like to talk to your employer or organization about

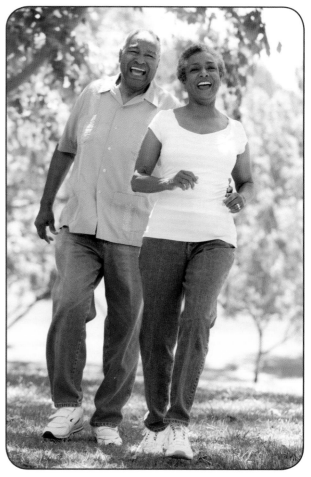

Start getting back to exercise as soon as you can after your treatment.

making your hours more flexible for a period before, during, and after treatment. In fact, I encourage most of my patients to get back to work if they want to during their radiation treatment. Some people find it difficult to talk with colleagues or friends about the experience of being diagnosed with DCIS. If you want to, share your experience with just a few close friends or colleagues. Sharing your feelings could give you valuable support.

Complementary Therapies

Complementary therapies are used by some women in addition to their regular treatments. For example, relaxation therapy can reduce anxiety and feelings of pain. Exercising can help you to feel less tired and can reduce your chance of weight gain. It's important to remember that many "natural" or "herbal" medications have not been proven to work, nor have they been tested for side effects or their interactions with regular treatments.

CONTROL POINT #18 – LIFE AFTER DCIS

WARNING

It takes time to get through the stress of a diagnosis of DCIS. Although it's precancerous, you will be mixing with patients with cancer. This can make you feel scared and sometimes even a little awkward because your disease has a much better prognosis.

TIP

Consider getting back to work and a regular exercise program as soon as you can.

REMEMBER

It's best to stop all hormonal contraception after being diagnosed with DCIS, and therefore sexual activity may become a problem. Talk to your doctors and nurses about your options for contraception. Communicate with your partner about sexual activity and intimacy.

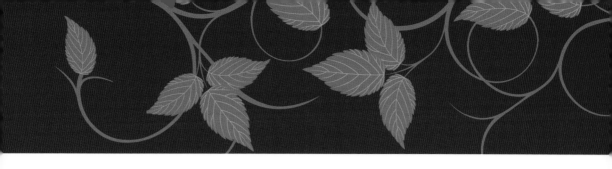

CONTROL POINT #19

WHAT CHECKS DO I NEED AFTER MY TREATMENT?

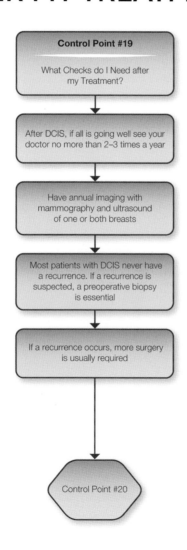

Control Point #19

What Checks do I Need after my Treatment?

↓

After DCIS, if all is going well see your doctor no more than 2–3 times a year

↓

Have annual imaging with mammography and ultrasound of one or both breasts

↓

Most patients with DCIS never have a recurrence. If a recurrence is suspected, a preoperative biopsy is essential

↓

If a recurrence occurs, more surgery is usually required

↓

Control Point #20

19

Having Checks after Your Treatment

Completing treatment is exciting but can also be stressful, particularly when the "umbilical cord" that had regularly linked you with your treatment team is suddenly cut. Having no more regular appointments sometimes increases fear and uncertainty.

It's only natural to feel this way, but it does get better with time. For now, it's important to go to all of your scheduled follow-up appointments after treatment; and if you're worried, don't hesitate to make an earlier appointment. It can be scary at first, so keep in touch with your treatment team and your general practitioner. Try to coordinate your visits so that you see a different member of your team every four to six months, rather than seeing more than one member of your team within a few weeks.

The frequency of follow-up visits varies from treatment center to treatment center. Most problems tend to occur in the first five years, so the frequency of checkups can be reduced to once per year after five years. You still need to have annual breast X-rays (Figure 19.1), and these may be followed up by an appointment with your family doctor.

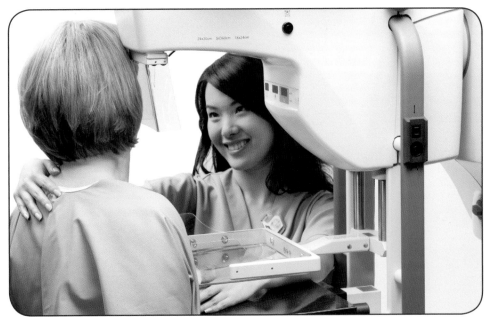

Figure 19.1 It is very important to have a mammogram and an ultrasound once a year after treatment.

Important aspects of follow-up include:

- Your doctor asking you if you have any symptoms from the disease or its treatment.

- Your doctor reviewing a mammogram with or without an ultrasound at every anniversary of your treatment.

- You or your doctor asking about any side effects from your surgery, radiation, or hormonal treatment.

- Your doctor performing a physical exam to look for any signs of recurrence or a new problem in your other breast. Your doctor should at least check under the armpits and above the collarbone area, the breast, and chest wall area.

- Organizing an annual mammogram and/or breast ultrasound of one (if you've had a mastectomy) or both sides (if you've had breast conservation). Perhaps they may also discuss the role of breast MRI.

- Having a yearly pelvic exam if you're taking tamoxifen because this drug can very slightly increase your risk of uterine cancer. The main way to detect this, however, is to watch for any unusual spotting, particularly after the menopause. Be sure to tell your doctor right away about any abnormal vaginal bleeding you may have.

- Remembering that most aches and pains are not cancer. You will get the odd back or muscle pain after gardening or exercise, or just sitting at your desk for a long time. Don't be afraid to take some Panadol or Tylenol and see if the pain goes away. If a new pain is persistent, make an earlier appointment for a checkup. Most of the time, pain will not be related to your cancer, but if you don't feel right, see your doctor. If a pain, lump, or other symptom persists, see your doctor.

- Maintaining your emotional and physical well-being. Look after your diet, keep exercising, and try not to put on too much weight.

- Remembering to have all your regular checks with your family doctor, including regular blood tests for diabetes, cholesterol, and so on.

Please try to get back to as much of your normal life and routine as possible. I know that's easier said than done, but there are some simple things you can do. Plan a weekend away, dates with your partner, and vacations with your family. Put off your doctors' appointments by a few weeks if they don't fit in with your vacation plans!

Recurrence after Breast Conservation without Radiation

If you have had a lumpectomy in the past for DCIS, it is very frustrating if your DCIS returns. You may have some regrets for not choosing a mastectomy or having radiation therapy after your initial lumpectomy. Hopefully, this will never happen to you. However, if it does occur, treatment can still be very successful. But let's try to "take control" again.

In many cases, it comes back in the same area of the breast. It is usually picked up on a mammogram as a new area of microcalcifications. If it is picked up as a lump, there is a chance that there may be areas of invasion present. In other words, it may have progressed to a real cancer. Here are the important steps:

1. Prove that it is a recurrence and not just benign calcification by having a core biopsy.

2. Ensure that you have an ultrasound of both breasts to check that there are no lumps (masses), which may indicate an invasive cancer as well as DCIS.

3. The next step is to determine whether it's pure DCIS, DCIS with possible invasion, or an invasive recurrence.

4. After determining that, the next question is whether the breast is potentially conservable again. If it is a small localized recurrence, then a breast MRI may help determine if there is more than one area.

5. If it is a solitary recurrence and can be removed with a margin of healthy breast, then a wide local excision is recommended if you still want to try to save your breast. If your doctor is not able to feel the area, then a hookwire localization may be required.

6. If it is a large area of pure DCIS (say greater than 30 mm), or there is microinvasion present, or it is an invasive recurrence, a sentinel node biopsy is also recommended.

7. If there is a malignant gland in the armpit, proved by needle biopsy, then it is an invasive recurrence and you will need some or all of the glands removed from the armpit as well as surgery to the breast.

8. If you need to have or choose to have a mastectomy on the side of the recurrence and if you have a very strong family history of breast cancer (which may have emerged after your original treatment) or the breast cancer gene, it may be worth having a discussion with your team about removing the other side as well. I'm not recommending this. It's just a good time to think about this difficult option.

9. Think about an immediate reconstruction after a mastectomy with an implant or flap type reconstruction.

10. If it is DCIS or an invasive recurrence and the margins are clear, then a course of radiation would be strongly recommended this second time around.

11. If you have an invasive recurrence, make sure the tumor is measured for estrogen and HER2 receptors.

12. If it is an invasive recurrence, make sure you see a medical oncologist to discuss the role, if any, for additional chemotherapy, Herceptin, or hormonal treatment.

Recurrence after Breast Conservation with Radiation

This is not common and, as mentioned in "Control Point # 14 – What Is My Prognosis?" most high-grade DCIS recurrences occur in the first five years after treatment, but low-grade DCIS can recur in between years five to ten also. Recurrences after ten years are less common.

There are a few important issues here. Follow the same advice as above for recurrence without radiation. The big differences here are:

1. For some patients with high-grade DCIS and treated by lumpectomy and radiation, the radiation can cause some "atypia" and even mimic a DCIS recurrence. For this reason, always proceed slowly and avoid having a **fine needle (aspiration) biopsy**, which just samples the cells; instead, always have a core biopsy to prove it is DCIS. Better still, have a wide local excision first if there is any doubt. Don't rush surgery if there is any doubt. I remember seeing a patient whose breast was removed at a small hospital by a general surgeon, after a "false-positive" DCIS recurrence after a fine needle biopsy.

2. Because you have already had radiation, the best treatment now is a total mastectomy.

3. As mentioned above, also think about whether it's time to have a mastectomy of the other side, particularly if you have a very strong family history of breast cancer.

4. Even though you have had radiation, sometimes it is still possible to insert an implant underneath your pectoral muscle. If this is not possible, consider a flap type reconstruction.

5. As above, see a medical oncologist if you have an invasive breast cancer to at least discuss the role of hormonal treatment or chemotherapy.

Recurrence of DCIS After a Mastectomy

This is very, very rare. If you find a lump under your scar or under the skin on the side of your mastectomy, insist on having a biopsy. If it proves to be an area of invasive breast cancer, have this widely excised. All other things being equal, I usually follow it up with radiation to the chest wall. If it's a large recurrence, there may be a case for removing some or all glands under your armpit and perhaps even having some chemotherapy or hormonal treatment.

A New Invasive Cancer or DCIS in the Other Breast

One of the reasons we do follow up with you after treatment is to make sure you don't get anything new in the other breast. In the NSABP B-17 study, the fifteen-year risk of developing a contralateral breast cancer was about 10% after a lumpectomy (with or without radiation) and 7% after lumpectomy, radiation, and tamoxifen.

There is no right or wrong answer as to how to treat the other side. You may have had a mastectomy on one side years and years ago; and for the new side, you decide to have breast conservation. Alternatively, for some women in this situation, I suggest having a mastectomy on the new side to balance things out (without further plastic surgery) or to take the opportunity, while under anesthetic, to have an implant inserted on both sides. This doesn't add too much to the operating time. Have a look at Pip's story on page 215.

Carol's Story

At the age of 48, happily married with a twenty-one-year-old son, a regular two-year mammogram detected DCIS in the right breast. I had been having mammograms every two years since I was 40 years of age. Not knowing much about breast cancer or having any family history that I knew of, my family and I were quite in shock. We were handed a lot of information (too much at the time). So much information at one time was very overwhelming.

After being referred to a breast cancer surgeon, it was decided that I'd undergo a lumpectomy. After all further testing was done, it was decided that no further treatment would be necessary because the DCIS was the smallest the surgeon had ever seen. Radiotherapy was discussed, but the doctors thought it would be an overkill of treatment.

Unfortunately, two years later the DCIS returned in the same breast and in the same area. I was devastated, not wanting to believe I would be going down the same path once again. Once again, it was very small, so I had another lumpectomy on the same day two years later! This time I decided to have radiotherapy.

With the support of my loving family and friends, I have now been eight years free of any DCIS or breast cancer. I have regular yearly checks and am optimistic that the cancer has gone forever.

Upon reflection, my decision to take responsibility for my ongoing health and having routine checkups has convinced me that my life now is very different than what it might have been if I had been diagnosed with a more advanced stage of breast cancer.

Pip's Story

I'd had tender, lumpy breasts most of my adult life. After routine mammograms and ultrasounds found cysts, I regularly had these aspirated by a surgeon in his rooms. He was great and very accurate in locating them, and I felt no pain. This continued for several years until another routine mammogram showed suspicious areas. A referral to a breast specialist confirmed widespread DCIS in the left breast and the need for a mastectomy. I opted for a latissimus dorsi flap with an implant done in conjunction with mastectomy. Unfortunately, infection meant removal of that implant, and I wore a heavy prosthesis for about six months until a new saline implant went in. It doesn't look good enough to go topless, but it gives me shape. I had total gland clearance and, therefore, I needed no chemo or radiation. I joined a gym to exercise and reduce risk of lymphedema, which never developed. That was in 1998. Routine mammograms afterwards always showed no significant change until thirteen years later when they saw one small, deep localized area of DCIS in the opposite right breast. This was fortunate as I had some choice of treatment. I opted for a wide excision of the DCIS (with clearance confirmed by pathology), followed by six weeks of radiation—the best option known for good results based on long-term studies. I am a nurse, and I have always been very positive. I have great trust and faith in our specialists. They have never let me down.

Staying Positive after a DCIS Recurrence

At this point you feel quite down. You may have been through all your treatment and the damn DCIS has come back. You may look back at some of your choices and have some regrets. I'd just like to say, it's best to look forward. The DCIS or invasive cancer may have come back in any case. Dust yourself off and face the new challenge. You've done it before, and I'm sure you can do it again.

CONTROL POINT #19 – WHAT CHECKS DO I NEED AFTER MY TREATMENT?

WARNING

Completing treatment is exciting but can also be stressful, particularly when the "umbilical cord" that had regularly linked you with your treatment team is suddenly cut. Having no more regular appointments sometimes increases fear and uncertainty.

TIP

See your doctor no more than twice a year to start with after treatment, and then once a year is all you need if all is well after your treatment of DCIS.

REMEMBER

If your disease comes back as pure DCIS again, treatment can be nearly 100% effective. If it comes back as invasive cancer and it has not spread to the lymph glands, the success rates in that situation are also high.

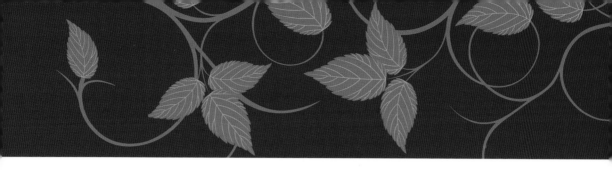

CONTROL POINT #20

IMPORTANT QUESTIONS FOR YOUR TREATMENT TEAM

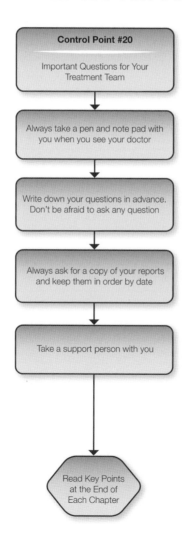

Control Point #20

Important Questions for Your Treatment Team

Always take a pen and note pad with you when you see your doctor

Write down your questions in advance. Don't be afraid to ask any question

Always ask for a copy of your reports and keep them in order by date

Take a support person with you

Read Key Points at the End of Each Chapter

20

I see patients who have no questions and others who have two to three pages of questions. From my perspective, it's important for a doctor or team to answer your questions. However, you should also be mindful of other patients waiting to see the doctor in the waiting room. If you have lots of questions, try calling the medical receptionist to get an extended appointment or see if you can be the last patient on the doctor's list or simply see the doctor on two separate visits. I remember one patient with DCIS who I saw weekly for 30 to 40 minutes for three weeks before she was comfortable to go ahead with radiation after surgical removal of her DCIS. Another trick you can use is to tell the doctor up front what your top 4 or 5 concerns are that you need sorted out at this particular clinic visit. This chapter contains a list of questions that can guide your thinking. Highlight the important ones for you before or after your surgery. A lot of the answers can, of course, be found in this book, so please don't hit your team with all of these questions! Also a lot of the answers can be found on the Web site of your team members, breast care nurse or other therapists.

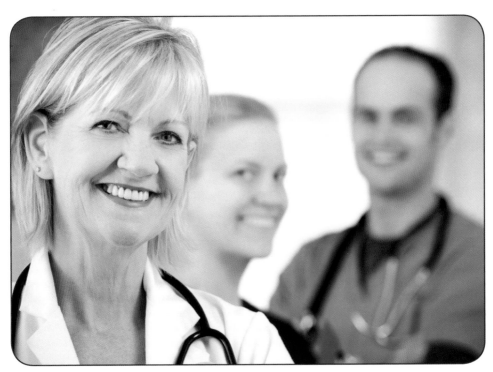

See your doctors regularly after treatment and don't hesitate to ask them questions.

Before Your Surgery

How sure are you that I have DCIS and not just hyperplasia?

How large is the area of DCIS on my mammogram?

Is the area of DCIS in more than one part of the breast (multicentric or multifocal)?

Do I need any tests before surgery? (Common tests are mammogram, ultrasound, and core biopsy.)

Do I need to have a breast MRI before my surgery? (This may be useful if you have dense breasts, if you have a strong family history of breast cancer, or Paget's disease of the nipple.)

Do I need to have a mastectomy (breast removal)?

Do I need a sentinel node biopsy? (I normally recommend this if you have a large area of DCIS over about 40 to 50 mm, or if there is any microinvasion on the preoperative core biopsy, or you are having a mastectomy and unsuspected invasive cancer may be found after your surgery.)

If I have a sentinel node biopsy, how is it mapped? When and where is this done?

If I have a sentinel node biopsy, will you do a quick test on it while I'm asleep to see if it's involved?

Where do I go to check in for my procedure?

How long do I fast before the surgery?

Can any of my medications increase the risk of side effects from my surgery?

Do you perform other types of surgery apart from breast surgery?

If I have breast conservation, how will you place the scar?

If I have a DCIS that has only been found on the mammogram and can't be felt, how do you remove it? (A localization procedure with a hookwire is usually required using a mammogram or ultrasound to insert a guide wire or other marker to the cancer.)

Can I see a radiation oncologist before my surgery?

Who is in your treatment team?

Will doctors who specialize in breast cancer treat me?

If I have a mastectomy, can I have an immediate reconstruction? If not, why not?

Are there any clinical research trials or studies I should know about?

How long will I be in the hospital?

Will I have a drain inserted into my incision?

Will I need to have stitches (sutures) removed after the surgery?

How long might it take me to recover from surgery?

How much will surgery cost? (Check the costs of others services associated with surgery, such as the anesthetic or pathology testing, etc.)

Will I have any pain with the treatment? What will be done about this?

Is there a financial gap between what the government/insurance pays and your fee?

Are there any side effects I should watch out for?

After Your Surgery

What type of DCIS do I have? (The common types are comedo, solid, papillary, or cribriform.)

Can I have a copy of my pathology report please?

What is the grade of my DCIS (1, 2, or 3)?

What is the size of my DCIS?

Is there calcification in the DCIS?

Is there any "necrosis" (cells that have died)? (Comedo-type necrosis is more significant than a few dead cells here and there.)

If there is calcification, is it in areas of DCIS? (often within areas of necrosis)

Are there any areas of true invasion or microinvasion?

Are my margins clear?

If yes, where is the closest margin, and how close in millimeters is the DCIS to that margin? (We like to see a 2 mm margin if possible.)

Is my tumor ER-positive?

Was my sentinel node involved?

Have the final tests (immunohistochemistry) come back on the sentinel node yet?

If the sentinel node is involved, how involved is it (isolated tumor cells, micrometastasis, or a larger macrometastasis)?

How many nodes were removed from my armpit?

Do I need any further surgery?

Do I need any further tests (such as an MRI or another mammogram)?

When will I see a radiation oncologist? Or do I need to see a radiation oncologist? If not, why not?

Do I need physical therapy (physiotherapy) for my shoulder?

When does my drain come out?

How do I take care of my arm?

When can I start to drive?

When can I go back to work?

I would like to have a second opinion. Can you refer me to someone else?

Are there any DCIS support groups who can help me?

About Your Radiation Therapy

Do I need radiation therapy?

Which areas of my breast will get radiation therapy? (usually all of it)

How long is the course of the radiation therapy?

Will I have to miss work?

What times is the radiation therapy department open?

How long does the radiation therapy planning session take to complete?

What should I bring with me to the radiation therapy planning session? (usually X-rays and maybe a consent form)

Is there any way to get help with traveling to and from the radiation therapy department?

Where do I park when I'm having radiation therapy?

Is there a fee for parking during radiation therapy?

How long is the wait before radiation starts after my radiation therapy planning session?

How many radiation therapy treatments will be given? (usually 15 to 30)

Will I need a radiation boost? (This is an extra dose to where the DCIS was originally found.)

What are the common side effects after radiation therapy?

What are the uncommon side effects after radiation therapy?

What are the long-term side effects after radiation therapy?

Who will talk to me about looking after my skin and avoiding these side effects?

How often will I be checked by you, your nurse, or radiation therapist while I'm having radiation therapy?

Is there a number I can call if I'm worried about anything during my radiation therapy?

Will the radiation therapy touch my heart?

Should I give up smoking or drinking during my radiation therapy? (It's normally a good idea to give up smoking.)

If I have radiation therapy to my chest wall, will it affect my chances of having a breast implant (reconstruction) later?

How long does each radiation treatment take while I'm under the machine? (Usually, the radiation is turned on for about fifty seconds in each treatment location.)

How long will I be in the radiation therapy department every day?

How much does radiation therapy cost, and will I get any rebates from the government or my insurance company?

About Hormonal Treatment

How do you decide if I need hormonal treatment for my DCIS?

What side effects might I have during and after my treatment?

What are the benefits of hormonal treatment for me?

How long should I take the hormonal treatment?

Are there any other drugs I can have instead of tamoxifen?

Do any of my other medications interfere with tamoxifen?

What time of day do I take my hormonal treatment?

Will tamoxifen stop my periods?

Is tamoxifen enough for contraception?

I've read about the new hormone therapies called aromatase inhibitors. Should I have these instead?

If I use aromatase inhibitors, will you check my bone density?

What are the main side effects of aromatase inhibitors?

Will you check my blood vitamin D levels?

About Your Checkups

Who should I see for my follow-up visits?

When do I see you again after my surgery and/or radiation?

When do I have my next mammogram?

Do I need a breast MRI?

Do I need a breast ultrasound?

How often do I need to come back for a follow-up check?

Who should I contact if I'm worried between my checks?

How do I look after my arm? (if you have had surgery to the axilla)

What do I do about contraception?

When can I have a baby?

I really wish you all the very best and hope that *DCIS of the Breast: Taking Control* has helped you. Don't hesitate to send me feedback via email at info@breastcancertakingcontrol.com.au or the breast cancer taking control Facebook page.

Remember to enjoy some of life's pleasures—reading, gardening, eating and drinking well, walking, music, traveling, loving, community, family, and friends. Life goes on after DCIS.

CONTROL POINT #20 – IMPORTANT QUESTIONS FOR YOUR TREATMENT TEAM

 WARNING Many patients find follow-up appointments stressful as they are a reminder of the challenges of treatment.

 TIP Take a list of your concerns that you want to discuss with your doctor and let them know what they are at the start of the consultation.

 REMEMBER There is no such thing as a silly question. If you're worried about anything at all, bring it to the attention of your doctor or nurse.

GLOSSARY

ABSCESS: A boil or collection of pus caused by infection.

ADJUVANT: Additional treatment given after surgery to increase the chances of survival, including hormonal treatment, chemotherapy, or radiation therapy.

AREOLA: The dark skin around your nipple.

AROMATASE: A special chemical in the body that produces estrogen after you have gone through menopause. Aromatase is part of a family of chemicals called enzymes.

AROMATASE INHIBITOR (AI): A drug that reduces the production of estrogen in the body after you have gone through menopause. Three drugs in this class are available: anastrozole (Arimidex), letrozole (Femara), and exemestane (Aromasin).

ATYPIA: A change in the lining of the ducts in your breast wherein they start to look "atypical" or abnormal. The medical terms include atypical ductal or atypical lobular hyperplasia.

AXILLA: The armpit.

AXILLARY CLEARANCE: Surgery that removes a fat pad from under your armpit that contains some or all of the lymph nodes.

AXILLARY DISSECTION: See "AXILLARY CLEARANCE"

BIOPSY: A test involving the removal of cells (fine needle biopsy) or tissue (core biopsy) for diagnosis.

BLOOD COUNT: A test that measures the number of red and white blood cells and platelets in your blood.

BONE SCAN: A type of X-ray scan where a small trace of radioactivity is injected into a vein in your arm and is then taken up by all your bones. Cancer appears as a "hot spot" or an abnormal area.

BOOST: An extra course of radiation to the tumor bed.

BRANCHING CALCIFICATIONS: A type of calcification often seen on a mammogram; it is caused by high-grade DCIS.

BRCA1 OR BRCA2 GENE: Human genes that belong to a class of genes known as tumor suppressors. Mutations or "defects" of these genes have been linked to hereditary breast and ovarian cancer.

BREAST CONSERVATION: See "LUMPECTOMY"

BREAST PROSTHESIS: An artificial breast or breast form, usually made of silicone gel, that can be worn inside your bra or inserted by a plastic surgeon permanently under your chest muscles (a breast implant) following a mastectomy.

CAPSULITIS: Thickening that can occur around an internal breast prosthesis or implant, particularly if radiation is given.

CASTING CALCIFICATIONS: A type of calcification often seen on a mammogram; it is caused by high-grade DCIS forming the perception of a "cast," similar to a plaster cast of the inside of the duct.

CATARACT: Clouding of the lens inside the eye.

CELLULITIS: A rapid onset, spreading infection of the deep tissues of the skin. This causes the skin to become hot and tender and may cause fever, chills, sweats, and swollen and tender nodes.

CENTRAL WEDGE EXCISION: Excision of the nipple, areola and underlying tissue, usually for Paget's disease.

CHEMOTHERAPY (chemo, cytotoxic drugs, anticancer drugs): The use of drugs, usually given intravenously, to kill, slow, or stall the growth of cancer cells.

CLAVICLE: The breastbone at the base of the neck.

CLINICAL TRIAL: Research, conducted with your permission, that usually involves a comparison of two or more treatments (an existing treatment is compared to a new and potentially better treatment). Which patients receive the old treatment and the new treatment is randomly allocated by a computer.

COLUMNAR CELL HYPERPLASIA: See "HYPERPLASIA"

COMEDO: An old term to describe a high-grade DCIS. It was first called this because of the cells dying in the center of the duct (see "NECROSIS"), liquefying, and then eventually calcifying.

COMEDONECROSIS: See "COMEDO"

CONTRALATERAL SYMMETRIZATION: Part of oncoplastic surgery, where symmetry of both breasts is achieved with a breast lift or "mastopexy" or a breast reduction of the opposite healthy side.

CORDING: An uncommon side effect after surgery appearing as a painful string-like tissue extending down the inner arm from the armpit to the hand. It is treated with vitamin E cream and massage.

CORE BIOPSY: The sampling of breast tissue with a needle larger than that used in a fine needle biopsy. A core biopsy produces a tiny cylinder or core of tissue for examination by a pathologist to work out whether a lump or abnormal mammogram could be cancer.

CT (COMPUTED TOMOGRAPHY) SCAN: An X-ray test taken from different angles of a part of the body. These images are combined by a computer to make cross-sectional pictures of your body. A contrast dye is sometimes injected to help blood vessels show up.

DEEP INFERIOR EPIGASTRIC PERFORATOR (DIEP) FLAP: A type of "free" tissue reconstruction that is not joined to the original donor site with a pedicle or fixed blood supply.

DELAYED RECONSTRUCTION: A surgical procedure performed to recreate a breast, done some time after the mastectomy treatment for breast cancer.

DENSITY: A term used to describe an abnormal, noncalcified area on a mammogram. The change often implies a mass (or breast lump) but may be due to normal glandular tissue.

DONOR SITE: The part of the body from where healthy tissue is moved to another part of the body (usually the chest wall) after a mastectomy.

DOSIMETRIST: A specially trained radiation therapist who calculates the angles and doses of the treatment prescribed by your radiation oncologist.

DUCTAL CARCINOMA IN SITU: See "DCIS"

DUCTOGRAM: An X-ray where radio-opaque dye is injected into a nipple duct to find a cause for discharging blood or fluid.

DUCTS: Tube-like passage that bring breast milk from the lobules to the nipple.

ENDOMETRIAL CANCER: Cancer of the womb.

ESTROGEN: A female hormone that is used in the brain and in female parts of the body such as the breast, womb, and vagina.

ESTROGEN RECEPTOR (ER): A type of antenna inside the nerve center or "nucleus" of a breast cancer cell or normal cell that binds to estrogen in the bloodstream and allows it to work inside the cell. If it is present it is called "ER-positive"; if absent, it is called "ER-negative."

EXTERNAL-BEAM RADIATION: Usually produced by a linear accelerator to kill cancer cells.

FALSE NEGATIVE: A test result (such as a sentinel node biopsy) that shows no cancer present when in fact you actually have cancer that went undetected.

FALSE POSITIVE: A test result (such as a sentinel node biopsy or mammogram) that shows a possible cancer present when in fact you actually don't have cancer.

FINE NEEDLE (ASPIRATION) BIOPSY: The sampling of breast tissue with a thin needle to suck out cells for examination by a pathologist using a microscope. It is not as accurate as a core biopsy, but it is quicker to perform and done using standard needles used for taking blood.

FIRST DEGREE RELATIVE: Includes parents, offspring, and siblings, but for DCIS it is usually your mother, sister, or daughter. But note, breast cancer and DCIS can occur in men.

FLAP RECONSTRUCTION: A breast reconstruction involving normal tissue from another part of the body that remains connected to the blood supply from the original or donor location by a flap or pedicle.

FRACTIONS: The daily doses of or attendance for radiation.

FREE FLAP: A type of flap reconstruction where the tissue is separated from the original donor site and reconnected to the chest area using microsurgery.

FROZEN SECTION: A quick method for a pathologist to examine possible cancerous tissue while you're asleep during surgery. This is often done on a sentinel node, but it's not routinely used except when a mastectomy is planned and a diagnosis has not been firmly established before your surgery.

GAMMA CAMERA: An X-ray machine that detects radioactive dye in a sentinel lymph node.

GENOTYPING: Working out the genetic makeup of an individual cell.

GLANDS: A term for lymph nodes surrounding your breast in the axilla, internal mammary chain, or supraclavicular fossa. See also "IMC" and "SCF"

GLUTEAL FLAP: A type of breast reconstruction that uses part of your buttock.

GOOGLE SCHOLAR: Part of Google that allows users to search for academic works.

GRADE: A measure of how slow (low-grade) or fast (high-grade) a cancer is growing. A grade 1 tumor is slower growing and looks more ordered under a microscope than a grade 3 tumor.

GRANULAR CALCIFICATIONS: Calcifications that are more circular than straight are often a sign of DCIS on a mammogram. They can be fine granular (usually fainter and smaller) or coarse granular (usually larger and easier to see).

GRAY (Gy): A dose unit of radiation therapy. One Gray = 100 rads. See "RAD"

HEMATOMA: A lump caused by a collection of blood beneath the skin, usually with a surrounding bruise.

HER2 RECEPTOR: A receptor on the surface of all cells known as a human epidermal growth factor receptor 2, which regulates the growth of cells. HER2 positivity or overexpression refers to having an excessive number of HER2 receptors on your breast cancer cells. This occurs in about one in three to one in four women with DCIS. The role of Herceptin for DCIS is still being investigated.

HERCEPTIN (TRASTUZUMAB): A drug used to bind to the HER2 receptor to prevent it from binding to circulating growth factors in the blood that can cause excessive cell growth.

HISTOLOGIC GRADE: See "GRADE"

HOOKWIRE: This involves inserting a guide wire via X-ray or, less frequently, ultrasound control and positioning it just beyond the abnormal area in your mammogram. Under anesthetic, the surgeon will follow the wire to find and remove the abnormality at the tip of the wire, along with a rim of surrounding healthy tissue, and then remove the wire with the piece of breast tissue attached.

HORMONAL TREATMENT: These are usually tablets that can block the effect of estrogen or lower estrogen levels to stop it stimulating the estrogen receptor often present within DCIS.

HORMONE POSITIVE: See "ESTROGEN RECEPTOR (ER)"

HORMONE REPLACEMENT THERAPY (HRT): Tablets taken to replace a woman's natural hormones after menopause. More recently has been called "hormone therapy" or "HT."

HYPERPLASIA: A change in the lining of the ducts in your breast where they increase in number and start to pile up on each other. It may occur in the duct (ductal hyperplasia) or the lobule (lobular hyperplasia) of the breast.

IMC: See "INTERNAL MAMMARY CHAIN"

IMMEDIATE RECONSTRUCTION: A surgical procedure or procedures performed to recreate a breast, done at the same time as a mastectomy.

IMMUNOHISTOCHEMISTRY (IHC) STAIN: A chemical stain used by a pathologist to work out whether a specific cell or receptor (such as HER2 or ER) is present in the tissue.

IMPLANT: See "BREAST PROSTHESIS"

IN-SITU HYBRIDIZATION (ISH) TEST: A more accurate test than the immunohistochemistry (IHC) test used to detect HER2. It takes one to two weeks to complete.

INFILTRATING DUCTAL CARCINOMA: The most common type of invasive breast cancer, wherein the cells have invaded or infiltrated through the breast duct wall. This is real cancer and not preinvasive or precancer like DCIS.

INFRAMAMMARY FOLD: Also known as the inframammary crease or inframammary line, this is the anatomical boundary of a breast from below where it meets the chest.

INTERNAL MAMMARY CHAIN (IMC): The lymph glands behind the breastbone or sternum where breast cancer can spread.

INVASIVE CARCINOMA: Cancer cells that have invaded through the duct or lobule of the breast.

INVASIVE LOBULAR CARCINOMA: The second most common type of breast cancer, which starts in the lobules of the breast where milk is normally made after pregnancy.

ISOLATED TUMOR CELLS (ITCs): Single cells or small clusters of cells not greater than 0.2 mm in largest dimension and classified as pN0(i) in an axillary sentinel node. These are usually not seen by the naked eye but picked up using specials stains or chemicals called immunohistochemistry (or IHC) stain.

KERATIN: A protein which makes up the outer layer of skin produced on top of the nipple when Paget's disease is present.

LANGER'S LINES: The natural lines or creases all over the skin. Surgical wounds made parallel to Langer's lines generally heal better and produce less scarring than those that are perpendicular or cut across Langer's lines.

LATISSIMUS DORSI MUSCLE FLAP: A tissue reconstruction using part of the muscle around your shoulder. Also called an "LD flap."

LINEAR ACCELERATOR: A machine that produces high-energy X-rays to destroy cancer cells. It can produce penetrating X-rays or less-penetrating electrons.

LINEAR CALCIFICATIONS: A type of calcification often seen on a mammogram usually associated with high-grade DCIS.

LIPOFILLING: The removal of fat tissue from another part of the body such as the tummy area, which is then injected into the reconstructed breast to improve its shape or fullness.

LOBULAR CARCINOMA IN SITU (LCIS): A condition in which abnormal cells are found in the lobules of the breast. Its name is misleading as this is not cancer but is a condition (not unlike having a family history) that has been shown to increase the risk of breast cancer in either breast in the future.

LOBULES: The "leaves" connected to the top of the breast ducts that expand and produce milk after pregnancy.

LOCAL RECURRENCE: Cancer coming back in the breast after breast conservation, or on the chest wall or surrounding lymph nodes after a mastectomy.

LUMPECTOMY: Surgical removal of a breast cancer with a healthy margin of normal breast; it is usually followed by radiation to the remaining portion of the breast.

LYMPH: Fluid composed of white cells, blood products, and digested food, which helps to fight infection. Lymph is carried throughout the body by the lymphatic system to the lymph glands.

LYMPH GLANDS: Tissues in the lymphatic system that act as filters to fight infection or cancer. These may be felt under the arm if you have breast cancer.

LYMPH NODES: See "LYMPH GLANDS"

LYMPH VESSELS: See "LYMPHATIC SYSTEM"

LYMPHATIC SYSTEM: Small vessels, called lymphatics, that carry lymph fluid all around the body, including the breast.

LYMPHEDEMA: Swelling of the arm after treatment to the armpit because of blocked lymphatics causing a backup of fluid.

LYMPHOSCINTIGRAPHY (LYMPHATIC MAPPING): The use of radioactive dye that is taken up by lymphatics and visible on a special camera called a gamma camera. This is done the night before or on the same day as a sentinel node biopsy.

MACROMETASTASES: Tumor deposits in a lymph node (gland) that are greater than 2.0 mm in dimension and easily visible without special IHC stains.

MACROSCOPIC REPORT: The part of your pathology report that describes what is seen by the pathologist with the naked eye before he or she cuts up the specimen and looks at your cancer with a microscope.

MAGNETIC RESONANCE IMAGING (MRI): An imaging test that uses strong magnets and radio waves to create pictures of the breast and surrounding tissue.

MAGNIFICATION VIEWS: Additional views using a mammogram machine to enlarge or magnify a suspicious area of calcification that may be DCIS.

MAMMOGRAM: A breast X-ray routinely done in two directions to characterize a lump, or as a screening test for breast cancer.

MARGIN: The edge of the tissue removed during a lumpectomy. A positive margin has DCIS extending to the edge.

MASTECTOMY: The surgical removal of your entire breast.

MEDICAL ONCOLOGIST: A doctor who specializes in treating cancer with chemotherapy drugs or hormone drugs.

MEDLINE: An electronic index of citations in medical journals from 1950 to the present, with a focus on the biomedical sciences.

META-ANALYSIS: A statistical method where the results of many smaller studies are lumped together to determine whether a specific treatment is beneficial or not.

METASTATIC DISEASE: Cancer that has spread beyond the breast and lymph glands to another part of the body.

MICROCALCIFICATION: Tiny deposits of calcium (as opposed to macrocalcifications, which are coarse calcium deposits) within the breast tissue. They are usually harmless, tiny specks of calcium, particularly when they are multiple; but when seen in one area, they are referred to as a cluster and may be an indicator of DCIS.

MICRODOCHECTOMY: Excision of an abnormal milk duct under an anesthetic.

MICROINVASION: One or more areas of invasive cancer penetrating the duct, generally measuring 1 mm or less, usually associated with high-grade DCIS.

MICROMETASTASES: Tumor deposits greater than 0.2 mm but not greater than 2.0 mm in dimension in the lymph nodes.

MICROSCOPIC REPORT: The part of your pathology report that describes what is seen by the pathologist when sections of your tumor are examined under magnification with a microscope.

MITOSIS: The process of cell division wherein one cells divides into two.

MITOTIC RATE: A measure taken into account when a tumor is graded, wherein the pathologist counts how many cells dividing into two he or she can see in your tumor.

MONDOR'S DISEASE: A thrombosed superficial vein of the breast that is linear and painful and may cause some indentation of the breast skin. Similar to cording.

MULTICENTRIC DISEASE: The presence of two or more areas of DCIS or cancer in different quadrants of the breast.

MULTIDISCIPLINARY TEAM: A team of doctors and other health care professionals who work and communicate with each other about the best possible treatment for your individual situation.

MULTIFOCAL DCIS: The presence of two or more areas of DCIS or cancer in the same quadrant of the breast.

MULTILEAF COLLIMATORS: The MLC is a specialized, computer-controlled device with as many as 160 Tungsten interdigitating leaves or fingers inside the linear accelerator allowing radiation beams to conform to the shape of the tumor. They allow radiation to be delivered in three dimensions to the breast but can block the radiation to normal structures such as the heart and lungs.

NECROSIS: This refers to the presence of cells that have become starved of oxygen and died, usually in the center of a duct full of DCIS.

NIPPLE-SPARING MASTECTOMY (NSM): The surgical removal of your entire breast whilst preserving the skin, nipple, and areola. This procedure leaves more skin behind than a total mastectomy.

NON-COMEDO: An older classification of DCIS that divided DCIS into two groups, comedo and non-comedo.

NODES: See "LYMPH GLANDS"

NUCLEOLUS: A small, round structure seen within the nucleus of the cell and thought to be important in producing protein.

NUCLEAR GRADE: This is how abnormal the nucleus (or control center) of the cancer cell looks. This is scored in a range from 1 to 3.

OCCULT DCIS: This is DCIS visible on magnetic resonance imaging (MRI) but not on a mammogram and ultrasound.

ONCOPLASTIC SURGERY: Combination of oncology (cancer specialty) and plastic surgery techniques usually by a breast surgeon who not only removes the cancer but works out how to maintain the look of the breast and its symmetry with the other side.

OSTEOPOROSIS: Weakening of the bones that occurs as you get older or from lack of estrogen due to menopause or drugs such as aromatase inhibitors.

PAGET'S DISEASE: A disease of the nipple usually associated with underlying DCIS or cancer.

PARTIAL BREAST IRRADIATION (PBI): A radiation technique where only the region surrounding the area where DCIS has been removed is irradiated to a high dose in a shorter period of time using a single dose of radiation at the time of surgery or after surgery by a radioactive wire or a linear accelerator. "See LINEAR ACCELERATOR"

PEDICLE FLAP: A piece of normal skin, fat and sometimes muscle moved from another part of the body to fill the defect left after a mastectomy.

PERIAREOLAR INCISION: Surgical removal of a breast tumor through a scar circularly placed around the areola. "See AREOLA"

PLASTIC SURGEON: A surgeon who specializes in breast reconstructive procedures.

POSTMASTECTOMY RADIATION THERAPY: The use of radiation to the chest wall and/or glands after a mastectomy.

PROGNOSIS: An estimation of the chance of DCIS returning in the breast as DCIS or as invasive cancer. It may also refer to the potential survival rate at a given point of time with or without treatment.

PRONE TABLE: A specially designed X-ray table where you lie facedown with your breast through a hole in the bed. A surgeon and/or radiologist performs the biopsy under the table using a digital X-ray of the abnormal area and software that calculates the exact location in three dimensions.

PUBMED: A Web site for finding the academic publications of your treating doctor.

RADIATION DOSE: See "GRAY"

RADIATION ONCOLOGIST: A doctor who specializes in treating cancer with radiation therapy. Also known as a radiotherapist.

RADIATION THERAPIST: A specially trained person who works the equipment that delivers radiation therapy.

RADIATION THERAPY (RADIOTHERAPY): The treatment of disease by radiation.

RADS: The imperial unit for a Gray. A common dose of radiation to the breast after removal of DCIS is 5000 rads, which is equivalent to 50 Gray.

REDUCTION MAMMOPLASTY: A plastic surgical procedure that reduces the size of your normal breast by removing skin, fat, and breast tissue. Always make sure that your surgeon sends the normal tissue for pathology testing.

SARCOMA: A type of cancer that forms from the surrounding or connective tissue such as muscle, fat, bone, cartilage, or blood vessels. A sarcoma occurs very rarely after treatment of breast cancer in a swollen arm or a breast previously treated with radiation.

SELECTIVE ESTROGEN RECEPTOR MODULATOR (SERM): A drug that acts like estrogen on some tissues but blocks the effect of estrogen on others. Tamoxifen (Nolvadex) and raloxifene (Evista) are two examples of SERMs.

SENTINEL NODE: A type of "guardian" lymph node through which the lymphatic vessels drain first before connecting to other lymph nodes. There are usually one to three sentinel nodes that drain each breast.

SENTINEL NODE BIOPSY: Removal of the sentinel node on the same side of the breast cancer after "sentinel node mapping"; and if that is clear, no further lymph nodes are taken.

SENTINEL NODE MAPPING: Identification of the sentinel lymph node(s) by injection of a radioactive substance, blue dye, or both near the tumor. A gamma camera is used to find the sentinel lymph node(s) before surgery with an X-ray. During surgery, the surgeon uses a probe to find the lymph node(s) containing the radioactive substance or looks for nodes which have stained blue. The surgeon then removes the sentinel node(s) to check for the presence of cancer either quickly while you are anesthetized ("quick-test") or thoroughly in the week after your surgery.

SEROMA: A short-lived fluid collection that occurs after surgery in your breast, chest wall, or armpit.

SEROUS FLUID: Straw-colored fluid that leaks from lymphatics and small blood vessels into tissues following surgery.

SIMULATION: A session where your radiation treatment setup is mocked up for your shape and size, and then a CT scan is done to map out your internal organs.

SKIN-SPARING MASTECTOMY (SSM): Mastectomy performed by removing the breast tissue through a small scar without removing all of the overlying skin. The natural shape and contour of the breast is recreated using either an implant or tissue flap. The nipple and areola are removed.

SPECIMEN X-RAY: An X-ray of your breast tissue removed usually using a needle localization procedure. This is to check that your DCIS (usually an area of calcifications) are not too close to the surgical cut edge. Also called a specimen radiograph.

STAGE 0, 1, 2, 3, 4: The degree of spread of all cancers is usually classified by four stages of increasing severity. For patients with breast cancer, stage 1 means that it is localized to the breast and stage 4 means that it has spread to other areas of the body. DCIS is sometimes called stage 0 (zero).

STEREOTACTIC BIOPSY: A biopsy procedure that uses a computer and X-ray guidance to insert a needle guided by a three-dimensional coordinate to obtain a fine needle or core biopsy of a breast abnormality and/or to insert a hookwire into the breast before surgery.

STERNUM: The breastbone.

SUB-CUTICULAR STITCHES: Dissolving sutures that are used to bring the skin together after surgery and are buried under the skin. They look and scar better than a "railroad track" type of stitch, which is external, needs removal, and leaves a more obvious scar.

SUPERFICIAL INFERIOR EPIGASTRIC ARTERY (SIEA) FLAP: A type of "free" tissue reconstruction wherein the tissue is not joined to the original donor site with a pedicle or fixed blood supply.

SUPRACLAVICULAR FOSSA (SCF): Lymph glands that are found just above the breastbone (clavicle).

SURGEON: A doctor who specializes in removing diseased tissue with surgery. Some surgeons are called surgical oncologists if they specialize in surgery for many cancers, or breast surgeons if they specifically specialize in breast cancer. Some surgeons are general surgeons, who may have an interest in breast cancer but may not necessarily work in a multidisciplinary team.

TAMOXIFEN: A drug that binds to estrogen receptors on cells to stop them from binding with circulating estrogen. Estrogen can make some breast cancer cells grow, and tamoxifen can starve these cells of estrogen and help them shrink or die.

TELANGIECTASIA: Prominent blood vessels that may appear in areas of skin that received a higher dose of radiation, such as over your scar or under your breast.

TERMINAL DUCT LOBULAR UNIT: The part of the breast duct that joins the lobule, which is thought to be where breast cancer usually begins.

THORACODORSAL ARTERY PERFORATOR FLAP (TAP FLAP): This is similar to a latissimus dorsi (LD) flap but it is "free-flap," requiring microsurgery to reconnect the blood vessels using a muscle and fat from near the shoulder blade.

TISSUE EXPANDER: A breast implant inserted under the skin and muscles of the chest; it is expanded over a few weeks by repeated injections of salt water (saline) to form a mound shaped like a breast after a mastectomy.

TOTAL MASTECTOMY: Removal of the entire breast without the underlying muscle or the lymph glands (lymph nodes) in the armpit (axilla).

TRANSVERSE RECTUS ABDOMINUS MUSCLE (TRAM) FLAP: A type of "pedicle" tissue reconstruction wherein the donor tissue is joined to the blood supply of the original donor site in the tummy area. By using tissue from your tummy, a "tummy tuck" is a bonus. Because it is fat and muscle, it feels more natural than an internal prosthesis or implant.

TUMOR BED: The area left behind after a cancer is removed; it is often at risk for cancer cells being left behind and therefore needs a higher dose of radiation, or a boost.

ULTRASOUND: High-frequency sound waves used to locate a tumor inside the body. A picture is shown on a computer or video screen, and it can show if a tumor is solid or contains fluid (a cyst).

VAN NUYS PROGNOSTIC INDEX (VNPI): Classification for DCIS based on nuclear grade, the presence or absence of necrosis, margin status and tumor size; originally thought to influence the chance of DCIS coming back after surgery.

USEFUL WEB SITES

Organization	Web site
American Cancer Society	www.cancer.org
Amoena—for breast styles and prostheses	www.amoena.com
American Society for Therapeutic Radiology and Oncology Patient Site	www.rtanswers.org
Australasian Lymphology Association	www.lymphoedema.org.au
Breastcancer.org	www.breastcancer.org
American Society of Clinical Oncology	www.plwc.org
Breast Cancer Care (U.K.)	www.breastcancercare.org.uk
Breast Cancer Network Australia	www.bcna.org.au
Cancer Australia	www.canceraustralia.gov.au In particular www.canceraustralia.gov.au/ publications-resources/cancer-australia-publications/ ductal-carcinoma-situ-dcis-understanding-your
Cancer Care	www.cancercare.org
Cancer Hope Network	www.cancerhopenetwork.org
Cancer Research UK	www.cancerhelp.org.uk
Clinical Trials (USA)	www.clinicaltrials.gov or www.centerwatch.com
ENCORE Gentle Exercise Program	www.ywca.org or www.ywcaencore.org.au
Intimacy Tips	www.breastcancer.org/tips/intimacy
Living Beyond Breast Cancer	www.lbbc.org
Look Good Feel Better	www.lookgoodfeelbetter.org or www.lookgoodfeelbetter.org.au
Lymphedema measurement	www.international.l-dex.com/what-is-l-dex
Macmillan Cancer Support	www.macmillan.org.uk

Organization	Web site
Memorial Sloan Kettering Cancer Center Recurrence Calculator	www.mskcc.org/APPLICATIONS/NOMOGRAMS/Breast/DuctalCarcinomaInSituRecurrencePage.aspx
My parent's cancer	www.myparentscancer.com.au/home.html
National Cancer Institute	www.cancer.gov/cancertopics/treatment/breast/surgerychoices
National Comprehensive Cancer Network	www.nccn.org
National Lymphedema Network	www.lymphnet.org
NEARLY ME® mastectomy products	www.nearlyme.org
Office of Cancer Complementary and Alternative Medicine	www.cancer.gov/cam/health_patients.html
Patient Advocate Foundation	www.patientadvocate.org
PubMed	www.ncbi.nlm.nih.gov/sites/entrez
Plastic Surgery	www.microsurgeon.org or www.bapras.org.uk
Quackwatch—Health-related frauds and myths	www.quackwatch.org
Resolve: The National Infertility Association	www.resolve.org
Radiological Society of North America (RSNA)	www.radiologyinfo.org
SHARE Cancer Support	www.sharecancersupport.org
Susan G. Komen Breast Cancer Foundation	www.komen.org
Understanding DCIS	www.dcis.info
Westmead Breast Cancer Institute (Australia)	www.bci.org.au
Women's Cancer Network	www.wcn.org
Young Survival Coalition	www.youngsurvival.org

CREDITS

Managing editors: Jess Ní Chuinn, Fiona Richardson

Cover: Shutterstock Images, under license:(Andrej Stojs) modified by Lorie De Worken: Mind the Margins

Internal book design: Astred Hicks: http://designcherry.com/ and Mishu Rahman (Shahanawaz A. Rahman)(including flow-charts): mishu@eyesometric.com

Copyeditor: Rachel Haimowitz

Proofreader: Laura Davies

Indexer: Russell Brooks

Preliminaries: iStockphoto, under license: "Debbie's Story" (PaulSimcock), Garden (Sternstunden), Shutterstock Images, under license: Rubik's cube (Mati Dovner) and by permission of Seven Towns Ltd; Dice (Chistoprudov Dmitriy Gennadievich), © BC Publishing Pty Ltd: Gum tree; Figures d,f (Margaret Mapperson), Key to Control Points (CP) and End of chapter symbols and Figure e (modified from Reference Going (2004)(© John Wiley & Sons Ltd by Mishu Rahman.

Chapter 1: iStockphoto, under license: Woman with left hand on cheek (MarsBars), © BC Publishing Pty Ltd: Figure 1.1 (Mishu Rahman), Figures 1.2–1.5, compliments of Prof. Michael Bilous, Healthscope Pathology; Figures 1.6, 1.7, 1.16, compliments of Dr Natacha Borecky, Westmead Breast Cancer Institute; Figure 1.8 © Siemens Healthcare; Figure 1.9 © Getty Images (BSIP) (Figures 1.10–1.15, with permission Prof John Boyages). Table 1.1, with permission: Wiley – International Journal of Cancer; Table 1.2: with permission LWW; Table 1.3 © 2004 de Roos et al; licensee BioMed.

Chapter 2: Figures 1.1–1.3 (compliments Google and PubMed.gov).

Chapter 3: iStockphoto, under license: children hugging (ejwhite), worried man (STEEX), Figures 3.1 (monkeybusinessimages).

Chapter 4: iStockphoto, under license; Figure 4.1, Rosebush, (nstanev); ©BC Publishing Pty Ltd: 4.2–4.4 (JazzIRT modified by Mishu Rahman); Figures 4.5-4.9; Figure 4.10 (with permission Dr. Elisabeth Elder).

Chapter 5: © BC Publishing Pty Ltd: Figure 5.6, Figures 5.1, 5.3–5.4 (Mishu Rahman); Figure 5.2 with permission of GE Healthcare © General Electric Company 2009; Figure 5.5 compliments A/Prof. Elizabeth Salisbury.

REFERENCES

Allred, D. C., Y. Wu, S. Mao, I. D. Nagtegaal, S. Lee, C. M. Perou, S. K. Mohsin, P. O'Connell, A. Tsimelzon, and D. Medina. 2008. Ductal carcinoma *in situ* and the emergence of diversity during breast cancer evolution. *Clinical Cancer Research* 14(2):370–378.

Ansari, B., S. A. Ogston, C. A. Purdie, D. J. Adamson, D. C. Brown, and A. M. Thompson. 2008. Meta-analysis of sentinel node biopsy in ductal carcinoma in situ of the breast. *British Journal of Surgery* 95:547–554.

Arias, E., B. L. Rostron, and B. Tejada-Vera. 2010. United States life tables, 2005. *National Vital Statistics Reports* from the Centers for Disease Control and Prevention, National Center for Health Statistics, National Vital Statistics System 58(10):1–132.

Aroner, S.A., Collins, L. C., Schnitt, S. J., Connolly, J. L., Colditz, G. A. and Tamimi, R. M.. 2010. Columnar cell lesions and subsequent breast cancer risk: A nested case-control study. *Breast Cancer Research* 12:R61.

Barreau, B., I. de Mascarel, C. Feuga, G. MacGrogan, M. H. Dilhuydy, V. Picot, J. M. Dilhuydy, C. T. de Lara, E. Bussières, and I. Schreer. 2005. Mammography of ductal carcinoma in situ of the breast: Review of 909 cases with radiographic-pathologic correlations. *European Journal of Radiology* 54:55–61.

Berger, J. C., and C. L. Clericuzio. 2008. Pierre Robin sequence associated with first trimester fetal tamoxifen exposure. *American Journal of Medical Genetics* Part A 146A:2141–2144.

Bijker, N., E. J. Rutgers, L. Duchateau, I. L. Peterse, J. P. Julien, and L. Cataliotti. 2001. Breast-conserving therapy for Paget disease of the nipple. A prospective European Organization for Research and Treatment of Cancer study of 61 patients. *Cancer* 91:472–477.

Bijker, N., P. Meijnen, J. L. Peterse, J. Bogaerts, I. Van Hoorebeeck, J. P. Julien, M. Gennaro, P. Rouanet, A. Avril, I. S. Fentiman, H. Bartelink, and E. J. Rutgers. 2006. Breast-conserving treatment with or without radiotherapy in ductal carcinoma-in-situ: Ten-year results of European Organisation for Research and Treatment of Cancer randomized phase III trial 10853—a study by the EORTC Breast Cancer Cooperative Group and EORTC Radiotherapy Group. *Journal of Clinical Oncology* 24:3381–3387.

Bloodgood, J. C. 1908. The clinical and pathological differential diagnosis of diseases of the female breast. *The American Journal of the Medical Sciences* 135:157–168.

Bober, S. L., A. Giobbie–Hurder, K.M. Emmons, E. Winer, and A. Partridge. 2013. Psychosexual functioning and body image following a diagnosis of ductal carcinoma in situ. *The Journal Of Sexual Medicine* 10:370–377.

Borud, E. K., T. Alraek, A. White, V. Fonnebo, A. E. Eggen, M. Hammar, L. L. Astrand, E. Theodorsson, and S. Grimsgaard. 2009. The Acupuncture on Hot Flushes Among Menopausal Women (ACUFLASH) study, a randomized controlled trial. *Menopause* 16:484–493.

Boyages, J., G. Delaney, and R. Taylor. 1999. Predictors of local recurrence after treatment of ductal carcinoma in situ: A meta-analysis. *Cancer* 85(3):616–28.

Broekhuizen, L. N., J. H. Wijsman, J. L. Peterse, and E. J. Rutgers. 2006. The incidence and significance of micrometastases in lymph nodes of patients with ductal carcinoma in situ and T1a carcinoma of the breast. *European Journal of Surgical Oncology* 32:502–506.

Bundred, N. J., A. Cramer, J. Morris, L. Renshaw, K. L. Cheung, P. Flint, R. Johnson, O. Young, G. Landberg, S. Grassby, L. Turner, A. Baildam, L. Barr, and J. M. Dixon. 2010. Cyclooxygenase-2 inhibition does not improve the reduction in ductal carcinoma in situ proliferation with aromatase inhibitor therapy: results of the ERISAC randomized placebo-controlled trial. *Clinical Cancer Research* 16:1605–1612.

Bur, M. E., M. J. Zimarowski, S. J. Schnitt, S. Baker, and R. Lew. 1992. Estrogen receptor immunohistochemistry in carcinoma in situ of the breast. *Cancer* 69:1174–1181.

Caliskan, M., G. Gatti, I. Sosnovskikh, N. Rotmensz, E. Botteri, S. Musmeci, G. Rosali dos Santos, G. Viale, and A. Luini. 2008. Paget's disease of the breast: The experience of the European Institute of Oncology and review of the literature. *Breast Cancer Research and Treatment* 112:513–521.

Cancer Research UK. http://info.cancerresearchuk.org/cancerstats/types/breast (accessed November 2010).

Carlson, G. W., A. Page, E. Johnson, K. Nicholson, T. M. Styblo, and W. C. Wood. 2007. Local recurrence of ductal carcinoma in situ after skin-sparing mastectomy. *Journal of the American College of Surgery* 204:1074–1080.

Carter, D. 1986. Margins of "lumpectomy" for breast cancer. *Human Pathology* 17:330–332.

Chen, C-Y., L. M. Sun, and B. O. Anderson. 2006. Paget disease of the breast: Changing patterns of incidence, clinical presentation, and treatment in the U.S. *Cancer* 107:1448–1458.

Chien, A. J., and P. E. Goss. 2006. Aromatase inhibitors and bone health in women with breast cancer. *Journal of Clinical Oncology* 24:5305–5312.

Chlebowski, R. T., and N. Col. 2012. Postmenopausal Women with DCIS Post–Mastectomy: A Potential Role for Aromatase Inhibitors. *The Breast Journal* 18(4):299–302.

Ciocca, R. M., T. Li, G. M. Freedman, and M. Morrow. 2008. Presence of lobular carcinoma in situ does not increase local recurrence in patients treated with breast-conserving therapy. *Annals of Surgical Oncology* 15:2263–227.

Claus, E. B., S. Petruzella, E. Matloff, and D. Carter. 2005. Prevalence of BRCA1 and BRCA2 mutations in women diagnosed with ductal carcinoma in situ. *Journal of the American Medical Association* 293(8):964–969.

Coombs, N. J., Cronin, K. A., Taylor, R. J., Freedman, A. N. and Boyages, J. 2010. The impact of changes in hormone therapy on breast cancer incidence in the US population. *Cancer Causes and Control* 21:83–90.

Cutuli, B., J. M. Dilhuydy, B. De Lafontan, J. Berlie, M. Lacroze, F. Lesaunier, Y. Graic, J. Tortochaux, M. Resbeut, T. Lesimple, E. Gamelin, F. Campana, M. Reme-Saumon, V. Moncho-Bernier, J. C. Cuilliere, C. Marchal, G. De Gislain, T. D. N'Guyen, E. Teissier, and M. Velten. 1997. Ductal carcinoma in situ of the male breast. Analysis of 31 cases. *European Journal of Cancer* 33:35–38.

Cutuli, B., C. Lemanski, A. Fourquet, B. de Lafontan, S. Giard, A. Meunier, R. Pioud-Martigny, F. Campana, H. Marsiglia, S. Lancrenon, E. Mery, F. Penault-Llorca, E. Fondrinier, and C. Tunon de Lara. 2009. Breast-conserving surgery with or without radiotherapy *vs* mastectomy for ductal carcinoma *in situ*: French Survey experience. *British Journal of Cancer* 100(7):1048–1054.

Cuzick, J., I. Sestak, S. E. Pinder, I. O. Ellis, S. Forsyth, N. J. Bundred, J. F. Forbes, H. Bishop, I. S. Fentiman, and W. D. George. 2011. Effect of tamoxifen and radiotherapy in women with locally excised ductal carcinoma in situ: Long-term results from the UK/ANZ DCIS trial. *The Lancet Oncology* 12:21–29.

Davies, C., H. Pan, J. Godwin, R. Gray, R. Arriagada, V. Raina, M. Abraham, V. H. Alencar, A. Badran, X. Bonfill, J. Bradbury, M. Clarke, R. Collins, S. R. Davis, A. Delmestri, J. F. Forbes, P. Haddad, M-F. Hou, M. Inbar, H. Khaled, J. Kielanowska, W-H. Kwan, B. S. Mathew, B. Müller, A. Nicolucci, O. Peralta, F. Pernas, L. Petruzelka, T. Pienkowski, B. Rajan, M. T. Rubach, S. Tort, G. Urrútia, M. Valentini, Y. Wang, and R. Peto. 2013. Long-term effects of continuing adjuvant tamoxifen to 10 years versus stopping at 5 years after diagnosis of oestrogen receptor-positive breast cancer: ATLAS, a randomised trial. *The Lancet* 381:805–816.

De Morgan, S., S. Redman, C. D'Este, and K. Rogers. 2011. Knowledge, satisfaction with information, decisional conflict and psychological morbidity amongst women diagnosed with ductal carcinoma in situ (DCIS). *Patient Education and Counseling* 84:62–8.

De Morgan, S., S. Redman, K. J. White, B. Cakir, and J. Boyages. 2002. "Well, have I got cancer or haven't I?" The psycho-social issues for women diagnosed with ductal carcinoma in situ. *Health Expectations* 5(4):310–318.

de Roos, M. A. J., R. M. Pijnappel, W. J. Post, J. de Vries, P. C. Baas, and L. D. Groote. 2004. Correlation between imaging and pathology in ductal carcinoma in situ of the breast. *World Journal of Surgical Oncology* 2.1:4. © 2004 de Roos et al; licensee BioMed Central Ltd. http://www.wjso.com/content/2/1/4.

Didier, F., D. Radice, S. Gandini, R. Bedolis, N. Rotmensz, A. Maldifassi, B. Santillo, A. Luini, V. Galimberti, E. Scaffidi, F. Lupo, S. Martella, and J. Y. Petit. 2009. Does nipple preservation in mastectomy improve satisfaction with cosmetic results, psychological adjustment, body image and sexuality? *Breast Cancer Research and Treatment* 118:623–633.

Dixon, A. R., M. H. Galea, I. O. Ellis, C. W. Elston, and R. W. Blamey. 1991. Paget's disease of the nipple. *British Journal of Surgery* 78:722–723.

Donker, M., S. Litière, G. Werutsky, J-P. Julien, I.S. Fentiman, R.A. Agresti, P. Rouanet, C. Tunon de Lara, H. Bartelink, N. Duez, E.J.T. Rutgers and N. Bijker. 2013. Breast-conserving treatment with or without radiotherapy in ductal carcinoma in situ: 15-year recurrence rates and outcome after a recurrence, from the EORTC 10853 randomized phase III trial. *Journal of Clinical Oncology* 31: 4054–4059.

Duffy, S. W., O. Agbaje, L. Tabar, B. Vitak, N. Bjurstam, L. Björneld, J. P. Myles, and J. Warwick. 2005. Overdiagnosis and overtreatment of breast cancer: Estimates of overdiagnosis from two trials of mammographic screening for breast cancer. *Breast Cancer Research* 7(6):258–265.

Dunne, C., J. P. Burke, M. Morrow, and M. R. Kell. 2009. Effect of margin status on local recurrence after breast conservation and radiation therapy for ductal carcinoma in situ. *Journal of Clinical Oncology* 27:1615–1620.

Durrieu, G., M. Rigal, R. Bugat, and M. Lapeyre-Mestre. 2004. Fertility and outcomes of pregnancy after chemotherapy in a sample of childbearing aged women. *Fundamental & Clinical Pharmacology* 18:573–579.

Early Breast Cancer Trialists' Collaborative Group (EBCTCG). 2010. Overview of the randomized trials of radiotherapy in ductal carcinoma in situ of the breast. *Journal of the National Cancer Institute Monographs* 41:162–177.

Evans, D. G., A. D. Baildam, E. Anderson, A. Brain, A. Shenton, H. F. Vasen, D. Eccles, A. Lucassen, G. Pichert, H. Hamed, P. Moller, L. Maehle, P. J. Morrison, D. Stoppat-Lyonnet, H. Gregory, E. Smyth, D. Niederacher, C. Nestle-Krämling, J. Campbell, P. Hopwood, F. Lalloo, and A. Howell. 2009. Risk reducing mastectomy: Outcomes in 10 European Centres. *Journal of Medical Genetics* 46:254–258.

Felson, D. T., and S. R. Cummings. 2005. Aromatase inhibitors and the syndrome of arthralgias with estrogen deprivation. *Arthritis and Rheumatism* 52:2594–2598.

Fisher, B., J. Dignam, N. Wolmark, D. L. Wickerham, E. R. Fisher, E. Mamounas, R. Smith et al. 1999. Tamoxifen in treatment of intraductal breast cancer: National Surgical Adjuvant Breast and Bowel Project B-24 randomised controlled trial. *The Lancet* 353(9169):1993–2000.

Fourquet, A., F. Campana, P. Vielh, P. Schlienger, D. Jullien, and J. R. Vilcoq. 1987. Paget's disease of the nipple without detectable breast tumor: Conservative management with radiation therapy. *International Journal of Radiation Oncology, Biology, Physics* 13:1463–1465.

Freedman, A. N., B. Yu, M. H. Gail, J. P. Costantino, B. I. Graubard, V. G. Vogel, G. L. Anderson, and W. McCaskill-Stevens. 2011. Benefit/risk assessment for breast cancer chemoprevention with raloxifene or tamoxifen for women age 50 years or older. *Journal of Clinical Oncology* 29:2327–2333.

Gao, X., S. G. Fisher, and B. Emami. 2003. Risk of second primary cancer in the contralateral breast in women treated for early-stage breast cancer: A population-based study. *International Journal of Radiation Oncology, Biology, Physics* 56:1038–1045.

Giuliano, A. E., L. McCall, P. Beitsch, P. W. Whitworth, P. Blumencranz, A. M. Leitch, S. Saha, K. K. Hunt, M. Morrow, and K. Ballman. 2010. Locoregional recurrence after sentinel lymph node dissection with or without axillary dissection in patients with sentinel lymph node metastases: the American College of Surgeons Oncology Group Z0011 randomized trial. *Annals of Surgery* 252(3):426–433.

Going, J. J., and D. F. Moffat. 2004. Escaping from flatland: Clinical and biological aspects of human mammary duct anatomy in three dimensions. *Journal of Pathology* 203:538–544.

Goldstein, N. S., F. A. Vicini, L. L. Kestin, and M. Thomas. 2000. Differences in the pathologic features of ductal carcinoma in situ of the breast based on patient age. *Cancer* 88:2553–2560.

Graham, R. A., M. J. Homer, J. Katz, J. Rothschild, H. Safaii, and S. Supran. 2002. The pancake phenomenon contributes to the inaccuracy of margin assessment in patients with breast cancer. *The American Journal of Surgery* 184:89–93.

Goss, P. E., Ingle J.N., Ales-Martinez, J.E., Cheung, A.M., Chlebowski, R.T., Wactawski-Wende, J., McTiernan, A. et al. for the NCIC CTG MAP.3. 2011 Study Investigators "Exemestane for breast-cancer prevention in postmenopausal women. *New England Journal of Medicine* 364:2381–2391.

Günhan-Bilgen, I., and A. Oktay. 2006. Paget's disease of the breast: Clinical, mammographic, sonographic and pathologic findings in 52 cases. *European Journal of Radiology* 60:256–263.

Harris, E. E., D. J. Schultz, C. A. Peters, and L. J. Solin. 2000. Relationship of family history and outcome after breast conservation therapy in women with ductal carcinoma in situ of the breast. *International Journal of Radiation Oncology, Biology, Physics* 48:933–941.

Ho, G.H., J. E. Calvano, M. Bisogna, P. I. Borgen, P. P. Rosen, L. K. Tan, and K. J. Van Zee. In microdissected ductal carcinoma in situ, HER-2/neu amplification, but not p53 mutation, is associated with high nuclear grade and comedo histology. *Cancer* 89:2153–2160.

Holland, R., J. H. Schuurmans Stekhoven, J. H. C. L. Hendriks, A. L. M. Verbeek, and M. Mravunac. 1990. Extent, distribution, and mammographic/histological correlations of breast ductal carcinoma in situ. *The Lancet* 335(8688):519–522.

Israel, P. Z., F. Vicini, A. B. Robbins, P. Shroff, M. McLaughlin, K. Grier, and M. Lyden. Ductal carcinoma in situ of the breast treated with accelerated partial breast irradiation using balloon-based brachytherapy. *Annals of Surgical Oncology* 17:2940–2944.

Jemal, A., R. Siegel, E. Ward, Y. Hao, J. Xu, and M. J. Thun. 2009. Cancer statistics, 2009. *CA: A Cancer Journal for Clinicians* 59:225–249.

Julian, T. B. 2011. A phase III clinical trial comparing trastuzumab given concurrently with radiation therapy and radiation therapy alone for women with HER2-positive ductal carcinoma in situ resected by lumpectomy: NSABP B-43. Abstract, San Antonio Breast Cancer Symposium, [OT10205].

Kendall, A., M. Dowsett, E. Folkerd, and I. Smith. 2006. Caution: Vaginal estradiol appears to be contraindicated in postmenopausal women on adjuvant aromatase inhibitors. *Annals of Oncology* 17:584–587.

Kenemans, P., N. J. Bundred, J. M. Foidart, E. Kubista, B. von Schoultz, P. Sismondi, R. Vassilopoulou-Sellin, C. H. Yip, J. Egberts, M. Mol-Arts, R. Mulder, S. van Os, and M. W. Beckmann. 2009. Safety and efficacy of tibolone in breast-cancer patients with vasomotor symptoms: A double-blind, randomised, non-inferiority trial. *The Lancet Oncology* 10:135–146.

Kennedy, F., D. Harcourt, and N. Rumsey. 2009. Perceptions of ductal carcinoma in situ (DCIS) among UK health professionals. *The Breast* 18:89–93.

Kennedy, S. H., B. S. Eisfeld, S. E. Dickens, J. R. Bacchiochi, and R. M. Bagby. 2000. Antidepressant-induced sexual dysfunction during treatment with moclobemide, paroxetine, sertraline, and venlafaxine. *Journal of Clinical Psychiatry* 61:276–281.

Kobraei, E. M., J. Nimtz, L. Wong, J. Buseman, P. Kemper, H. Wright, and B. D. Rinker. 2012. Risk factors for adverse outcome following skin-sparing mastectomy and immediate prosthetic reconstruction. *Plastic and Reconstructive Surgery* 129:234e–241e.

Kroman, N., M. B. Jensen, M. Melbye, J. Wohlfahrt, and H. T. Mouridsen. 1997. Should women be advised against pregnancy after breast-cancer treatment? *The Lancet* 350:319–322.

Krychman, Michael L. 2009. *100 questions & answers about women's sexual wellness and vitality: A practical guide for the woman seeking sexual fulfillment.* Boston: Jones and Bartlett.

Kuerer, H. M., C. T. Albarracin, W. T. Yang, R. D. Cardiff, A. M. Brewster, W. F. Symmans, N. M. Hylton, L. P. Middleton, S. Krishnamurthy, G. H. Perkins, G. Babiera, M. E. Edgerton, B. J. Czerniecki, B. K. Arun, and G. N. Hortobagyi. 2008. Ductal carcinoma in situ: State of the science and roadmap to advance the field. *Journal of Clinical Oncology* 27:279–288.

Kuhl, C. K., S. Schrading, H. B. Bieling, E. Wardelmann, C. C. Leutner, R. Koenig, W. Kuhn, and H. H. Schild. 2007. MRI for diagnosis of pure ductal carcinoma in situ: A prospective observational study. *The Lancet* 370:485–492.

Lagios, M. D., P. R. Westdahl, F. R. Margolin, and M. R. Rose. 1982. Duct carcinoma in situ. Relationship of extent of noninvasive disease to the frequency of occult invasion, multicentricity, lymph node metastases, and short-term treatment failures. *Cancer* 50:1309–1314.

Ligibel, J. A., A. Partridge, A. Giobbie-Hurder, M. Golshan, K. Emmons, and E. P. Winer. 2009. Physical activity behaviors in women with newly diagnosed ductal carcinoma-in-situ. *Annals of Surgical Oncology* 16:106–112.

Luo, J., Cochrane, B. B., Wactawski-Wende, J., Hunt, J. R., Ockene, J. K., & Margolis, K. L. (2013). Effects of menopausal hormone therapy on ductal carcinoma in situ of the breast. *Breast Cancer Research and Treatment* 137(3):915–925.

Marchal, C., B. Weber, B. de Lafontan, M. Resbeut, H. Mignotte, P. P. du Chatelard, B. Cutuli, M. Reme-Saumon, A. Broussier-Leroux, G. Chaplain, F. Lesaunier, J. M. Dilhuydy, and J. L. Lagrange. 1999. Nine breast angiosarcomas after conservative treatment for breast carcinoma: A survey from French Comprehensive Cancer Centers. *International Journal of Radiation Oncology, Biology, Physics* 44:113–119.

Marshall, J. K., K. A. Griffith, B. G. Haffty, L. J. Solin, F. A. Vicini, B. McCormick, D. E. Wazer, A. Recht, and L. J. Pierce. 2003. Conservative management of Paget disease of the breast with radiotherapy: 10- and 15-year results. *Cancer* 97:2142–2149.

Montague, E. D. 1984. Conservation surgery and radiation therapy in the treatment of operable breast cancer. *Cancer* 53:700–704.

Morrell, S., A. Barratt, L. Irwig, K. Howard, C. Biesheuvel, and B. Armstrong. 2010. Estimates of overdiagnosis of invasive breast cancer associated with screening mammography. *Cancer Causes & Control* 21:275–282.

Morrow, M. 2012. Refining the use of endocrine therapy for ductal carcinoma in situ. *Journal of Clinical Oncology* 30(12):1249–1251.

Mourits, M. J. E., E. G. E. de Vries, K. A. ten Hoor, A. G. J. van der Zee, and P. H. B. Willemse. 2007. Beware of amenorrhea during tamoxifen: It may be a wolf in sheep's clothing. *Journal of Clinical Oncology* 25:3787–3788.

Niraula, S., A. Ocana, M. Ennis, and P. J. Goodwin. 2012. Body size and breast cancer prognosis in relation to hormone receptor and menopausal status: A meta-analysis. *Breast Cancer Research and Treatment* 134:769–781.

Omlins, A., M. Amichetti, D. Azria, B. F. Cole, P. Fourneret, P. Poortmans, D. Naehrig, R. C. Miller, M. Krengli, C. Gutierrez Miguelez, D. Morgan, H. Goldberg, L. Scandolaro, P. Gastelblum, M. Ozsahin, D. Dohr, D. Christie, U. Oppitz, U. Abacioglu, G. Gruber, 2006. Boost radiotherapy in young women with ductal carcinoma in situ: a multicentre, retrospective study of the Rare Cancer Network. *Lancet Oncology* 7(8):652–656.

Pae, C. U., T. S. Kim, K. U. Lee, J. J. Kim, C. U. Lee, S. J. Lee, C. Lee, and H. H. Paik. 2005. Paroxetine-associated spontaneous sexual stimulation. *International Clinical Psychopharmacology* 20:339–341.

Paget, J. 1874. On the disease of the mammary areola preceding cancer of the mammary gland. *St. Bartholomew's Hospital Reports* 10:87–89.

Pandey, S., M. J. Kornstein, W. Shank, and E. S. de Paredes. 2007. Columnar cell lesions of the breast: Mammographic findings with histopathologic correlation. *Radiographics* 27(Suppl 1):79–89.

Partridge, A., J. P. Winer, M. Golshan, J. R. Bellon, E. Blood, E. C. Dees, E. Sampson, K. M. Emmons, and E. Winer. 2008. Perceptions and management approaches of physicians who care for women with ductal carcinoma in situ. *Clinical Breast Cancer* 8(3):275–280.

Patani, N., and K. Mokbel. 2008. Oncological and aesthetic considerations of skin-sparing mastectomy. *Breast Cancer Research and Treatment* 111:391–403.

Peled, A.W., R. D. Foster, A. C. Stover, K. Itakura, C. A. Ewing, M. Alvarado, E. Shelley Hwang, and L. J. Esserman. 2012. Outcomes after total skin-sparing mastectomy and immediate reconstruction in 657 breasts. *Annals Of Surgical Oncology* 19(11):3402–3409.

Petit, J. Y., E. Botteri, V. Lohsiriwat, M. Rietjens, F. De Lorenzi, C. Garusi, F. Rossetto et al. 2012. Locoregional recurrence risk after lipofilling in breast cancer patients. *Annals of Oncology* 23(3):582–588.

Pommier, P. et al. 2004. Phase III randomized trial of calendula officinalis compared with trolamine for the prevention of acute dermatitis during irradiation for breast cancer. *Journal of Clinical Oncology* 22:1447–1453.

Rashtian, A., S. Iganej, I. L. Amy Liu, and S. Natarajan. 2008. Close or positive margins after mastectomy for DCIS: Pattern of relapse and potential indications for radiotherapy. *International Journal of Radiation Oncology, Biology, Physics* 72:1016–1020.

Recht, A. 2009. Contralateral prophylactic mastectomy: Caveat emptor. *Journal of Clinical Oncology* 27:1347–1349.

Reeves, G. K., V. Beral, J. Green, T. Gathani, and D. Bull. 2006. Hormonal therapy for menopause and breast-cancer risk by histological type: A cohort study and meta-analysis. *The Lancet Oncology* 7:910–918.

Regolo, L., B. Ballardini, E. Gallarotti, E. Scoccia, and V. Zanini. 2008. Nipple sparing mastectomy: An innovative skin incision for an alternative approach. *Breast* 17:8–11.

Rosai, J. 1991. Borderline epithelial lesions of the breast. *The American Journal of Surgical Pathology* 15:209–221.

Rusby, J. E., E. F. Brachtel, M. Othus, J. S. Michaelson, F. C. Koerner, and B. L. Smith. 2008. Development and validation of a model predictive of occult nipple involvement in women undergoing mastectomy. *The British Journal of Surgery* 95:1356–1361.

Rusby, J. E., B. L. Smith, and G. P. Gui. 2010. Nipple-sparing mastectomy. *The British Journal of Surgery* 97:305–316.

Sackey, H., K. Sandelin, J. Frisell, M. Wickman, and Y. Brandberg. 2010. Ductal carcinoma in situ of the breast. Long-term follow-up of health-related quality of life, emotional reactions and body image. *European Journal of Surgical Oncology (EJSO)* 36(8):756–762.

Sanders, M. E., P. A. Schuyler, W. D. Dupont, and D. L. Page. 2005. The natural history of low-grade ductal carcinoma in situ of the breast in women treated by biopsy only revealed over 30 years of long-term follow-up. *Cancer* 103:2481–2484.

Sasano, H., Y. Miki, R. Shibuya, and T. Suzuki. 2010. Aromatase and in situ estrogen production in DCIS (ductal carcinoma in situ) of human breast. *Journal of Steroid Biochemistry & Molecular Biology* 118:242–245.

Schnitt, S. J., Connolly, J. L., Tavassoli, F. A., Fechner, R. E., Kempson, R. L., Gelman, R., & Page, D. L. 1992. Interobserver reproducibility in the diagnosis of ductal proliferative breast lesions using standardized criteria. *The American Journal of Surgical Pathology* 16:1133–1143.

Shugg, D., V. M. White, P. R. Kitchen, M. Pruden, J. P. Collins, and D. J. Hill. 2002. Surgical management of ductal carcinoma in situ in Australia in 1995. *ANZ Journal of Surgery* 72:708–715.

Silverstein, M. J., D. N. Poller, J. R. Waisman, W. J. Colburn, A. Barth, E. D. Gierson, B. Lewinsky, P. Gamagami, and D. J. Slamon. 1995. Prognostic classification of breast ductal carcinoma in-situ. *The Lancet* 345:1154–1157.

Smith, B. D., D. W. Arthur, T. A. Buchholz, B. G. Haffty, C. A. Hahn, P. H. Hardenbergh, T. B. Julian, L. B. Marks, D. A. Todor, F. A. Vicini, T. J. Whelan, J. White, J. Y. Wo, and J. R. Harris. 2009. Accelerated partial breast irradiation consensus statement from the American Society for Radiation Oncology (ASTRO). *International Journal of Radiation Oncology, Biology, Physics* 74:987–1001.

Smith, I. E., M. Dowsett, Y. S. Yap, G. Walsh, P. E. Lønning, R. J. Santen, and D. Hayes. 2006. Adjuvant aromatase inhibitors for early breast cancer after chemotherapy-induced amenorrhoea: Caution and suggested guidelines. *Journal of Clinical Oncology* 24:2444–2447.

Solin, L. J. 2010. The impact of adding radiation treatment after breast conservation surgery for ductal carcinoma in situ of the breast. *Journal of the National Cancer Institute Monographs* 41:187–192.

Solin, L., R. Gray, F. L. Baehner, S. Butler, S. Badve, C. Yoshizawa, S. Shak, L. Hughes, D. Page, G. Sledge, N. Davidson, E. A. Perez, J. Ingle, J. A. Sparano, and W. Wood. 2011. A quantitative multigene RT-PCR assay for predicting recurrence risk after surgical excision alone without irradiation for ductal carcinoma in situ (DCIS): A prospective validation study of the DCIS score from ECOG E5194. Abstract, San Antonio Breast Cancer Symposium [S4–6].

Solin, L. J., S. G. Orel, W. T. Hwang, E. E. Harris, and M. D. Schnall. 2008. Relationship of breast magnetic resonance imaging to outcome after breast-conservation treatment with radiation for women with early-stage invasive breast carcinoma or ductal carcinoma in situ. *Journal of Clinical Oncology* 26:386–391.

Stuart, K. E., N. Houssami, R. Taylor, and J. Boyages. 2011. Long-term outcomes of ductal carcinoma in situ of the breast: A systematic review and meta-analysis. *International Journal of Radiation Oncology, Biology, Physics* 81(2): S32.

Szelei-Stevens, K. A., R. R. Kuske, V. A. Yantsos, G. J. Cederbom, J. S. Bolton, and B. B. Fineberg. 2000. The influence of young age and positive family history of breast cancer on the prognosis of ductal carcinoma in situ treated by excision with or without radiation therapy or by mastectomy. *International Journal of Radiation Oncology, Biology, Physics* 48:943–949.

Taghian, A., M. Mohiuddin, R. Jagsi, S. Goldberg, E. Ceilley, and S. Powell. 2005. Current perceptions regarding surgical margin status after breast-conserving therapy: Results of a survey. *Annals of Surgery* 241:629–639.

Tokin, C., A. Weiss, J. Wang-Rodriguez, and S. L. Blair. 2012. Oncologic safety of skin-sparing and nipple-sparing mastectomy: A discussion and review of the literature. *International Journal of Surgical Oncology* Vol. 2012, Article ID 921821, 8 pages, 2012.

Torresan, R. Z., C. C. dos Santos, H. Okamura, and M. Alvarenga. 2005. Evaluation of residual glandular tissue after skin-sparing mastectomies. *Annals of Surgical Oncology* 12:1037–1044.

Toth, B. A., and P. Lappert. 1991. Modified skin incisions for mastectomy: The need for plastic surgical input in preoperative planning. *Plastic and Reconstructive Surgery* 87:1048–1053.

Tunon-de-Lara, C., I. de-Mascarel, G. Mac-Grogan, E. Stöckle, O. Jourdain, V. Acharian, C. Guegan, A. Faucher, E. Bussieres, M. Trojani, F. Bonichon, B. Barreau, M. H. Dilhuydy, J. M. Dilhuydy, L. Mauriac, M. Durand, and A. Avril. 2001. Analysis of 676 cases of ductal carcinoma in situ of the breast from 1971 to 1995: Diagnosis and treatment—the experience of one institute. *American Journal of Clinical Oncology* 24:531–536.

Tuttle, T. M., S. Jarosek, E. B. Habermann, A. Arrington, A. Abraham, T. J. Morris, and B. A. Virnig. 2009. Increasing rates of contralateral prophylactic mastectomy among patients with ductal carcinoma in situ. *Journal of Clinical Oncology* 27:1362–1367.

van Deurzen, C. H., M. de Boer, E. M. Monninkhof, P. Bult, E. van der Wall, V. C. Tjan-Heijnen, and P. J. van Diest. 2008. Non-sentinel lymph node metastases associated with isolated breast cancer cells in the sentinel node. *Journal of the National Cancer Institute* 100:1574–1580.

van la Parra, R. F., M. F. Ernst, P. C. Barneveld, J. M. Broekman, M. J. Rutten, and K. Bosscha. 2008. The value of sentinel lymph node biopsy in ductal carcinoma in situ (DCIS) and DCIS with microinvasion of the breast. *European Journal of Surgical Oncology* 34:631–635.

Velpeau, Alfred. 1856. *A treatise on cancer of the breast and of the mammary region.* Translated from the French by W. Marsden, M.D. London: Henry Renshaw, 356, Strand. Digitized by Google Books (http://books.google.com).

Verkooijen, H. M. 2002. Diagnostic accuracy of stereotactic large-core needle biopsy for nonpalpable breast disease: Results of a multicenter prospective study with 95% surgical confirmation. *International Journal of Cancer* 99:853–859.

Visvanathan, Kala, Patricia Hurley, Elissa Bantug, Powel Brown, Nananda F. Col, Jack Cuzick, Nancy E. Davidson et al. 2013. Use of Pharmacologic Interventions for Breast Cancer Risk Reduction: American Society of Clinical Oncology Clinical Practice Guideline. *Journal of Clinical Oncology* 31(23): 2942–2962.

Vogel, V. G., J. P. Costantino, D. L. Wickerham, W. M. Cronin, R. S. Cecchini, J. N. Atkins, T. B. Bevers, L. Fehrenbacher, E. R. Pajon, J. L. Wade III, A. Robidoux, R. G. Margolese, J. James, C. D. Runowicz, P. A. Ganz, S. E. Reis, W. McCaskill-Stevens, L. G. Ford, V. C. Jordan, and N. Wolmark. 2010. Update of the national surgical adjuvant breast and bowel project study of tamoxifen and raloxifene (STAR) P-2 trial: Preventing breast cancer. *Cancer Prevention Research* 3:696–706.

Waddell, B. E., P. C. Stomper, J. L. DeFazio, T. C. Hurd, and S. B. Edge. 2000. Postexcision mammography is indicated after resection of ductal carcinoma-in-situ of the breast. *Annals of Surgical Oncology* 7:665–668.

Wai, E. S., Lesperance, M. L., Alexander, C. S., Truong, P. T., Culp, M., Moccia, P., Lunqvist J.F. and Olivotto, I. A. 2011. Effect of radiotherapy boost and hypofractionation on outcomes in ductal carcinoma in situ. *Cancer* 117(1):54–62.

Wapnir, I. L., J. J. Dignam, B. Fisher, E. P. Mamounas, S. J. Anderson, T. B. Julian, S. R. Land, R. G. Margolese, S. M. Swain, J. P. Costantino, and N. Wolmark. 2011. Long-term outcomes of invasive ipsilateral breast tumor recurrences after lumpectomy in NSABP B-17 and B-24 randomized clinical trials for DCIS. *Journal of the National Cancer Institute* 103:478–488.

Warren, J. C. 1907. Abnormal involution of the mammary gland, with its treatment by operation. *The American Journal of the Medical Sciences* 133:521–534.

Wells, W. A., P. A. Carney, M. S. Eliassen, M. R. Grove, and A. N. Tosteson. 2000. Pathologists' agreement with experts and reproducibility of breast ductal carcinoma-in-situ classification schemes. *The American Journal of Surgical Pathology* 24(5):651–659.

Whelan, T. J., Pignol, J. P., Levine, M. N., Julian, J. A., MacKenzie, R., Parpia, S. and Freeman, C. 2010. Long-term results of hypofractionated radiation therapy for breast cancer. *New England Journal of Medicine* 362(6):513–520.

Wijayanayagam, A., A. S. Kumar, R. D. Foster, and L. J. Esserman. 2008. Optimizing the total skin-sparing mastectomy. *Archives of Surgery* 143:38–45.

Zafrani, B., A. Fourquet, J. R. Vilcoq, M. Legal, and R. Calle. 1986. Conservative management of intraductal breast carcinoma with tumorectomy and radiation therapy. *Cancer* 57:1299–1301.

INDEX

MY THOUGHTS AND NOTES

Write down your thoughts, feelings, or questions here, in the margins of the book or consider getting a journal or start a blog. Sometimes writing down your worries helps you to work through them. Don't forget to have a glass of champagne or your favorite drink when you have finished your treatment. Stand tall and move forward.

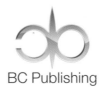

BC Publishing

Publisher of high quality books to help you Take Control after a cancer diagnosis

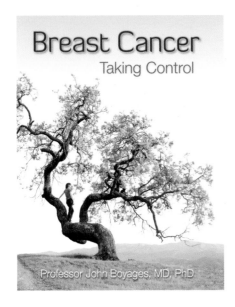

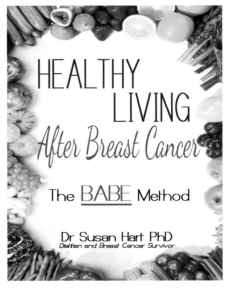

Coming Soon

Male Breast Cancer: Taking Control

an Ebook by Prof John Boyages

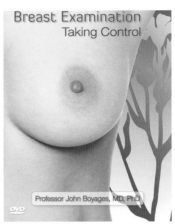